Cardiovascular Fluid Dynamics

Author
Uri Dinnar, Ph.D.
Senior Lecturer
Department of Biomedical Engineering
Technion
Israel Institute of Technology
Haifa, Israel

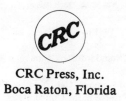

CRC Press, Inc.
Boca Raton, Florida

Library of Congress Cataloging in Publication Data

Dinnar, Uri.
Cardiovascular fluid dynamics.

  Bibliography: p.
  Includes index.
  1. Hemodynamics. I. Title.
QP105.D56   599.01'1   80-39565
ISBN 0-8493-5573-7

   Direct all inquiries to CRC Press, Inc., 2000 N.W. 24th Street, Boca Raton, Florida 33431.

International Standard Book Number 0-8493.5573-7

Library of Congress Card Number 80-39565
Printed in the United States

THE AUTHOR

Uri Dinnar is a senior lecturer at the Department of Biomedical Engineering at the Technion-Israel Institute of Technology at Haifa.

Dr. Dinnar obtained his undergraduate training at the Technion in the Department of Mechanical Engineering receiving the B.Sc. degree in 1964. He continued his studies at Harvard University in Cambridge, Massachusetts, in the Division of Engineering and Applied Physics, receiving his M.Sc. in 1966 and Ph.D in 1969.

Upon the completion of his studies he returned to the Technion and assumed his present position.

From 1966 to 1968 he served as a visiting associate professor at Michigan State University.

Dr. Dinnar is a member of the IEEE, the Cardiovascular System Dynamics Society, and the International Federation of Engineering in Medicine and Biology.

His major current research interests relate to the flow of blood in converging elastic and tapered vessels and the formation of thrombi.

WITH LOVE AND RESPECT

to

Rachel and Arieh
Gottesdiener

Eyouna and Ephraim
Taiber

TABLE OF CONTENTS

Chapter 10
Fluid Mechanics of Thrombus Formation 215

Chapter 1

THE CARDIOVASCULAR BED AS A SYSTEM

A scientific approach to the flow of blood in the cardiovascular system comprises the study of a multiphenomena that necessitates the cooperation of scientists from almost the entire spectrum of science. The nature of problems encountered in the cardiovascular system includes the study of fluid flow, elastic and viscoelastic behavior of cardiac muscles and blood vessel wall, control of biological reference values and hemostasis, signal transmission and signal processing by body requirement and environmental condition, and many more. This partial list explains the complexity of considering the cardiovascular system as a lumped-parameters integrated system. Although the cardiovascular system is in no way linear, the only way to understand the contribution of each of these mechanisms to the complex reaction that takes place under a variety of circumstances, is to try and study each of these systems separately, and hope that science will one day be able to combine the separate subsystems into one unified system. There are many different ways to study the behavior of the cardiovascular system, and each one of them contains most or all of these disciplines. All of these different approaches are utilized in one way or another in the daily clinical routine of patients' diagnosis and prognosis.

A. The Whole Body as a Single Unit

The consideration of the entire human body as a single unit with a variable number of inputs and a final number of measurable outputs is the most usable model of the cardiovascular system in clinics today. For each input there is a different empirical transfer function, usually combined with an assumption that there is no interaction with other inputs. This is the basic approach underlying the clinical screaning of patients for the existance of problems in the cardiovascular system. An example for this type of modeling is the "treadmill test." In this test an external requirement of work load combined with a controlled environment are the inputs into the system (Figure 1). The most commonly used outputs for this test are the blood pressure, heart rate, and electrical activity of the heart. In this case the transfer function is not defined explicitly, but the evaluation of normal and abnormal is based on the empirical range of the output. Thus, ignoring all the other contributors to variations in output, the value of this output for various workloads determines the body response. If deviations from normal are significant, further tests are required to diagnose the origin, or origins, of the problem.

Similar models are used in blood glucose tolerance tests, where an input of food intake, usually glucose, is empirically compared with the measured level of sugar in the blood. In some cases, the input is not a controlled or even a measurable parameter, but a deviation from normal in the output parameter indicates a change in the parameter, or even the existance of such an input as is the case in white blood cell count as indicative output to an input condition of inflammation.

B. Single Organ as a Unit

When information about the characteristics of an organ is required for a better understanding of its function or behavior under various circumstances, this organ can be modeled as a unit by itself, with its own inputs and outputs. In doing so, the other organs and the rest of the cardiovascular system is omitted and changes in input values due to changes in other organs are ignored. Yet the organ is assumed to maintain all of its control functions, even when they actually come from other centers, for example, the central nervous system. Each of the body organs can be singled out to serve as the

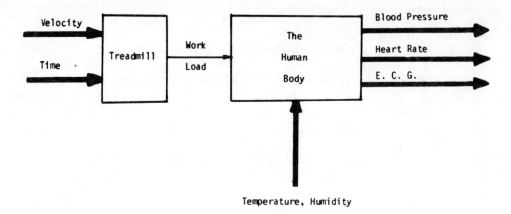

FIGURE 1.   Schematic diagram of the input and output parameters in the "treadmill test."

best such example. The heart can be considered as two pumps in series for the task of elevating blood pressure from the venous low pressure to arterial high pressure. While doing so, the heart must supply enough blood output to answer the demand of the entire circulation. The multiplication of the difference between arterial and venous pressure with the cardiac output gives the load of the heart, and can serve as a good indicative measure of heart condition. In this case the load of the heart is the independent variable, which describes the response of the heart to variable input conditions. Hence the heart is singled out as independent of the rest of the circulation. In the same way the lungs, situated between the two heart pumps, can be considered as a single unit by monitoring input and output respiratory parameters like inhaled and exhaled air composition and flow rates. By measuring the arterial and venous oxygen contents the two units can be combined to form a single unit comprising the heart and lungs. It is however, more appropriate to keep each one of them as a single unit and to form a lumped-parameter model with different inputs and different outputs at different locations (Figure 2). This model can be expanded by adding additional units to represent different organs in the human body, as discussed in the following chapters.

This model is of utmost importance in clinical use to evaluate the functioning of organs where further division of the system is too dangerous, i.e., the brain and the placenta in pregnant women. In the first case, further division is possible if a non-invasive technique is being used, like radioactive tracers. However, in the latter case, even these methods are incapable of supplying more detailed information.

C. Regions within a Single Organ

As was mentioned before it is possible to study only a segment of the brain as part of, or as independent of, the rest of the brain. This is most applicable to the diagnosis of pathology in a specific region, or for the effects of certain activity or drugs on this segment. Another example, discussed in detail in the text, is the study of the left ventricle. In this case the mechanisms of cardiac muscle contractions and the resulting pressure elevation and flow are combined to form a model of the left ventricle as a single unit separated from the rest of the circulation. The only connection to the remaining circulation is the ventricle filling and the aortic root pressure. This also is true in the study of heart valves, described in the appropriate chapter, where the elastic properties of the cusps control the opening of the valve, the flow formation, and the net amount of cardiac output. The reader will find out later that combining these two models into a lumped model is either too complex to yield some workable criteria, or can be achieved only with numerous simplifications so that very little information can be gained.

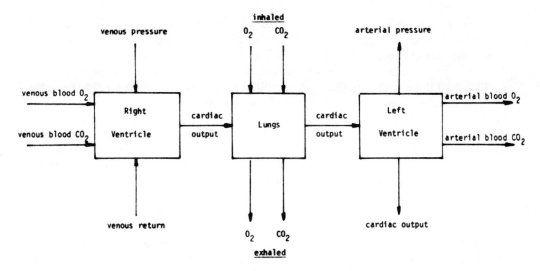

FIGURE 2.   Lumped-parameter model of the heart and lungs.

D. Part of the Arterial Tree

Because of the nature of the arterial tree, the flow of blood in arteries can not be studied as uniform for the entire circulation. The arterial tree, going down form the root of the aorta to the capillaries in the various organs and in the peripheral circulation, passes along its way blood vessels of varying cross-section and with different viscoelastic properties. Naturally the velocity and pressure distributions are different in different arterial segments. In addition, there is a continuous branching of the blood vessels which makes the analysis for more than a single branch very complex. The only way to study the transfer of mass along the circulatory tree is by study of a specific segment. This is important for the clinical measurements of rate of flow in a specific segment by noninvasive techniques, like radioactive tracers or ultrasonic Doppler. An accurate measurement requires the knowledge of velocity distribution at a given cross-section. It is also required in the study of local control mechanism, flow disturbances due to geometric constraints, and more. In the latter case, the flow disturbances can cause thrombus formation within the blood vessel. In this case the distribution of blood particles is essential to the understanding of thrombosis mechanisms together with the nature of mechanical interactions between the vessel wall and the various blood constituents. It is also important in the study of mechanical interactions between the different blood particles and between similar particles.

In the capillaries, where the actual transfer of oxygen to the tissues takes place, the study of flow rate and pressures must be combined with the study of fluid transport across the vessel walls. Thus, even if one arterial segment is considered, there is more than one measurable parameter.

In most published works the arterial segments are considered in isolation from the rest of the circulation. They are assumed to be far away from the branching sites, so that the entry effect can be ignored. The inflow is assumed known, so that outflow and fluid transport across the wall are obtained as a function of geometric changes and the mechanical properties of the segment wall.

E. Single Cells

Isolation of a single cell, and assuming the cell to represent a single system, means not only a change in scale, but mainly a change in approach. Three different phenomena must be considered: mechanical, electrical, and chemical. The mechanical system links the external stress conditions on the surface of the cells to the flow conditions in the vessels. Due to the shear stresses the cell will deform, roll, and move in prescribed direction. The deformation depends on the elastic properties of the cell that are associated with the chemical composition of the cell. This phenomena is of utmost importance in the flow through the microcirculation where the vessel diameter may be smaller than the cell size. In this case a significant deformation is required to push the cell through the capillary. The electrical phenomena is associated with the electric surface charge. The net charge on a platelet surface is negative. This negative charge attracts a layer of opposite charge around the surface and forms a double layer around the surface of the particle. The balance between the repulsion forces due to this electric charge and the van der Waals' forces of attraction is the main determinant of blood coagulation and the formation of thrombus.

Interactions with the blood vessel walls are determined by these forces: the mechanical repulsion force between particle and wall and the surface electric potential (zeta potential) of the wall surface. The chemical phenomena is divided into two separate mechanisms. The relation between external and internal concentration of different molecules determines the relative viscosity of the cell, the strength of the double layer, and the elasticity of the cell. This mechanism, controlled mainly by diffusion, is important in the determination of flow parameters. The other mechanism is the oxygen-hemoglobin reactions which are the main factor in the phenomena of oxygen transfer through the cardiovascular system, and in the supply of oxygen to the tissues. All these phenomena are related to each other in a very complicated way that is not completely understood. This makes the modeling of a single cell as a separate system very difficult. Because of this reason most of the work dealing with this subject had ignored one or two of the three mechanisms and studied the contribution of only one mechanism.

In the following chapters all of these models will be discussed in detail. Whenever possible integration of models to a larger model will be attempted.

Chapter 2

ELEMENTS OF PHYSIOLOGY OF THE CIRCULATORY SYSTEM

A. Introduction

This chapter does not intend, by any means, to cover the whole field of cardiovascular physiology. The main emphasis will be on the physical nature of the hydrodynamic problems associated with blood flow and fluid transfer. The physical aspects of blood flow will be summarized with the intention of supplying the required background for understanding the various systems described in the text, from a hydrodynamic point of view.

This chapter approaches the physiological mechanisms from a macroscopic point of view, and avoids, wherever possible, the considerations of various processes that take place on the level of cells. Hence, for example, the central nervous system is considered as a "black box" control mechanism. Processes of information transfer in and out of this box are considered without details of the actual cell-to-cell transfer mechanism.

The concentration, in this chapter, is on the phenomenological behavior of the cardiovascular system and on the description of its physical properties. For further reference the reader is advised to use the following books: Rushmer,[7] Burton,[1] and Ruch and Patton.[6] A reader with engineering background will find the book by Talbot and Gessner[8] closer to his interpretation of system analysis.

B. Structure and Function of the Systemic Circulation

The circulation of blood in the human body can be separated into two major systems. The pulmonary circulation initiates at the right ventricle and transmits blood only to the lungs, where filtration of CO_2 and supply of fresh oxygen take place. The systemic circulation which initiates the left ventricle is responsible for the supply of fresh blood to all the organs and tissues of the body, and thus can be considered as the feeding line of all the elements of the body. It is therefore logical to start the discussion by considering the peripheral circulation, which is the essential part of the systemic circulation.

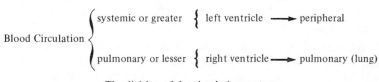

The division of the circulation system

The peripheral circulation must supply every single cell in the body with its necessary requirement of oxygen, metabolic fuel, vitamins, hormones, and heat. It also must remove heat and other waste products produced by the cell. To accomplish these functions, the blood supply to every single cell has to be in accordance with its individual needs, both in nutrition and the maintenance of heat balance. Since these requirements vary with activity, change in environmental conditions, excitement, and more, the circulation needs a very effective and sensitive control mechanism and the ability to increase or decrease flow into every small segment all over the body.

A reasonable question that can be asked now is *why circulation?* In single cell organisms the control requirements are so little that the constant supply of oxygen as well as waste removal is accomplished by a passive process of convection and free diffusion. This mechanism will not be discussed here. In mammals this process is carried out through the capillary walls, again mainly by free diffusion. Hence, all duties of the circulatory system are carried out at the capillary level. To supply each capillary according to its instantaneous needs and its function, requires an enormous number of control stations and an enormous number of routes for the passage of blood.

A survey of the literature will reveal two different approaches to the control process in the circulatory system. One, used mostly by engineers and system analysts, attributes the control characteristics to the larger blood vessels. The other, used mostly by biophysicists and biochemists, assigned to the capillaries and the single cells the same control properties. These two ideas will be analyzed and compared in the appropriate chapters. However, to shed some light on the nature of this control mechanism, some very elementary models can be used.

First Model

Assume that all the blood is condensed into a single elastic sphere. The diameter of the sphere is such that its volume equals the total volume of the blood vessels in the human body. Since total blood vessels volume is 5 l, this will correspond to a sphere diameter of 10.6 cm. The total blood volume in the human blood is 7 l. Squeezing this amount into the sphere will inflate the sphere, and will result in an increase in pressure inside the sphere.

Assume that the sphere is elastic and use Laplace's law to calculate the pressure inside the sphere, one obtains the following relations:

$$F = P \cdot \pi r^2 = \sigma \cdot 2\pi rt = E \frac{\Delta r}{r} 2\pi rt \qquad (1)$$

Hence

$$P = 2E \frac{\Delta r \cdot t}{r^2} \qquad (2)$$

where F is force, P the internal excessive pressure, r the sphere radius, σ the tension within the wall of the sphere, t the thickness of the wall, and E is the Young's modulus of the sphere material. After filling the sphere with blood there is an increase in radius, Δr. For explanation of all the terms defined in this case the reader is referred to Figure 1. Using an average value for Young's modulus (3×10^7 dyn/cm^2) and for the wall thickness (t = 0.12r), Equation 2 can be used to give a pressure of 20 mmHg. This part of the blood pressure is produced by the vessels of the cardiovascular system, all pressures in excess of this value are produced by the heart, which works as a pressure pump.

Second Model

Let's consider a pump in series with a closed tubing system, Figure 2. The tube may be rigid or flexible, and the flow rate through the tube equals the amount flowing in the systemic circulation. Consider the pressure on both sides of the pump to equal those of the average arterial (high) pressure and the average venous (low) pressure in the systemic circulation. The Poiseuille flow relations (Appendix 1) for viscous fluid flowing in a tube, may be employed to calculate the relation between length and radius required.

$$Q = \Delta P \cdot \frac{\pi r^4}{8\mu L} \qquad (3)$$

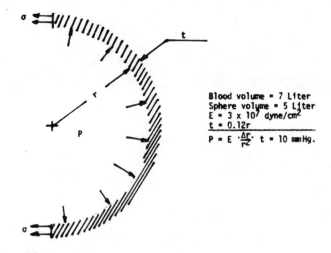

FIGURE 1. The elastic sphere model.

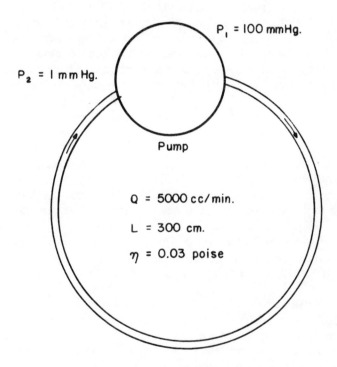

FIGURE 2. The single tube model.

where Q is the flow rate, ΔP the pressure drop, r the radius of the tube, L the tube length, and μ the fluid viscosity. For a required length of 300 cm, as an example, the required radius is 5.1 mm, so that a very compact tubing system is sufficient. The complexity of the actual system is therefore not due to hydrodynamic requirement, but rather due to various control functions and oxygen and metabolic nutrition supply. These requirements are thus essential and of utmost significance in the analysis of the geometry and bifurcation of the cardiovascular system.

Each component of the cardiovascular system can be described by its resistance to flow, R, defined by the linear relations:

$$Q = \frac{\Delta P}{R} \qquad\qquad (4)$$

When Poiseuille flow takes place, the resistance is given by:

$$R = \frac{8\mu L}{\P r^4} \qquad\qquad (5)$$

Hence the resistance depends on both the geometry of the blood vessels and the viscosity of the flowing blood. In physiology it is common to measure this resistance by Peripheral Resistance Units (PRU) defined as: *1 PRU is the resistance to a flow of 1 cc/min under a pressure of 1 mmHg.*

Administration of certain types of drugs (vasodilators) can increase the cross-sectional area of the blood vessels, hence decreasing their resistance. While by administration of others (vasoconstrictors), the cross-sectional area decreases and the resistance increases. Therefore, the resistance can serve as an indicator for the effectiveness of drugs, by measuring the flow rate, Q, and the pressure gradient, ΔP, before and after the administration of the drug, and computing an index for drug effectiveness.

The following tables give a summary of the average quantities of blood flow to various organs and tissues. All the tables refer to an average value under normal conditions. Most of these values will change under pathological conditions.

Table 1 gives the blood flow and oxygen consumption of different organs and tissues under normal conditions. Some conclusions can be interpreted from this table.

1. Oxygen consumption per gram of tissue can not serve, by itself, as an indicator for the requirement of blood flow to this tissue, since the tissue function might override this demand. For example, the blood flow to the kidney and liver is much larger than that defined by oxygen consumption, because of its function in the filtration of the blood.
2. Table 2 gives the calculated values for tissue and organ resistances. It is clear from this table that there is not any tissue or organ that can be singled out as having the major resistance, and thus serving as the main control of blood circulation. It should be noted that venous blood still contains nearly 75% of the arterial oxygen content. Hence, only 25% of the oxygen content of the arterial blood is being utilized by the tissues.

Since oxygen consumption and the value of the resistance of each organ and tissue are not sufficient for the definition of a control center, it is appropriate to try and divide the circulatory system according to some other criteria. This criteria can be the size of the blood vessels. Table 3 gives the diameter, length and cross-sectional area for the various vessels in the mesenteric vascular bed of the dog. Table 4 gives the appropriate parameters for an average human, and the calculated relative resistance and capacity for each diameter, based on Poiseuille's law. The following conclusions can be written from this table,

1. The highest resistance to flow lies in the arterioles and capillaries. So it is logical to assume that most of the control of blood flow is to be carried out at these locations. And in fact this is true, by vasoconstriction and vasodilation mechanisms the resistance will change and hence blood flow to either a specific organ or to the whole circulatory system. In addition to this vasomotor control there is an additional mechanism that is unique to the arterioles - capillaries interfaces.

Table 1
BLOOD FLOW AND OXYGEN CONSUMPTION OF DIFFERENT ORGANS AND TISSUES (AVERAGE VALUES UNDER NORMAL CONDITIONS)

Organ or Tissue	Mass (kg)	Blood flow			Oxygen consumption		
		ml/min	ml/min/100 g	% of total	ml/min	ml/min/100 g[a]	% of total
Liver	2.8	1375	49.1	27.5	51	1.82	20
Kidneys	0.3	1150	383.0	23	18	6.00	7
Skeletal muscle	34.0	750	2.2	15	50	0.15	20
Brain	1.5	700	46.6	14	46	3.07	18
Skin	3.6	300	8.3	6	12	0.33	5
Bones	23.0	250	1.1	5	35	0.15	14
Heart muscle	0.3	200	66.6	4	30	10.00	12
All others	4.5	275	6.1	5.5	8	0.18	3
Whole body	70.0	5000	7.1		250	0.36	

[a] Values are per 100 g of wet tissue.

Table 2
RELATIVE RESISTANCE OF DIFFERENT ORGANS AND TISSUES (AVERAGE VALUES UNDER NORMAL CONDITIONS)

Organ or Tissue	Blood flow ml/min	Relative resistance	Peripheral resistance units (dyn−sec/cm⁵) × 10⁻²
Liver	1375	3.6	2.9
Kidneys	1150	4.3	3.4
Skeletal muscle	750	6.6	5.3
Brain	700	7.1	5.7
Skin	300	16.6	13.3
Bones	250	20.0	16.0
Heart muscle	200	25.0	20.0
All others	275	18.1	14.5
Total	5000 ml/min		8000 dyn−sec/cm⁵

Table 3
MESENTERIC VASCULAR BED OF DOG

Kind of vessel	Diameter (mm)	Number	Length (cm)
Aorta	10	1	40
Large arteries	3	40	20
Main artery branches	1	600	10
Terminal branches	0.6	1,800	1
Arterioles	0.02	40,000,000	0.2
Capillaries	0.008	1,200,000,000	0.1
Venules	0.03	80,000,000	0.2
Terminal veins	1.5	1,800	1
Main venous branches	2.4	600	10
Large veins	6.0	40	20
Vena cava	12.5	1	40

From Middlemen, S., *Transport Phenomena in the Cardiovascular System*, Interscience, New York, 1976, 6. With permission.

Table 4

RELATIVE RESISTANCE AND CAPACITANCE OF VARIOUS BLOOD
VESSELS (BASED ON POISEUILLE'S LAW)

Kind of vessel	Average lumen diameter	Approximated total cross sectional area (cm²)	Percentage of blood volume contained		Relative capacity (%)	Relative resistance (%)
Aorta	2.5 cm	4.5	3 ⎫		4.5	4
Artery	0.4 cm	20	8 ⎬ 14		12.0	21
Arteriole	30 μm	400	3 ⎭		4.5	27
Capillary	6 μm	4500	4		6.0	41
Venule	20 μm	4000	4 ⎫		6.0	4
Vein	0.5 cm	40	12 ⎬ 49		18.0	1.5
Vena cava	3 cm	18	33 ⎭		49.0	1.5

It is the precapillary sphincter that upon contraction can reduce or even shut off
the flow into any capillary.

2.   The major part of the system capacitance is in the venous system. Hence changes
in total blood volume will be accommodated by the veins. This is achieved by
adjusting the total capacitance of the veins, a mechanism which is highly important in maintaining constant right atrial and right ventricle pressure under various
kinds of conditions.

An empirical expression for the branching of the blood vessels as described in Table
4 is given by:

$$A_i = 1.26 \, A_o \tag{6}$$

where A_o is the cross-sectional area of the mother vessel, and A_i total cross-sectional
area of the new generation. After n branching the total area is given by:

$$A_j = (1.26)^n \, A_o \tag{7}$$

Although these relations are very crude, they might be very useful for various calculations.

Figure 3 gives a general description of the blood route from the high pressure side
(aorta) to the low pressure side (vena cava). It can be seen from this figure that along
some of the branches there is a perfusion of only one capillary bed, while along other
branches there are two capillary beds in series (kidney) or even more (gastrointestinal
tract). This will require a more sophisticated control system, however, all of the routes
are in parallel and the influence of one of the others is therefore minor. In addition to
the branches shown in the figure there are thousands of other routes, some of them
are a direct connection between the high and low pressure side of the circulation system. These routes are called arteriovenous shunts, and will be discussed in a separate
chapter.

Table 5 summarizes the important physical properties of the cardiovascular system
that are essential for analytical treatment. Some of them will be discussed further in
the following chapters.

C. The Heart and the Cardiac Cycle

A schematic representation of the human heart chambers and the flow connections
are shown in Figure 4. The blood, rich in oxygen, leaves the heart through the left

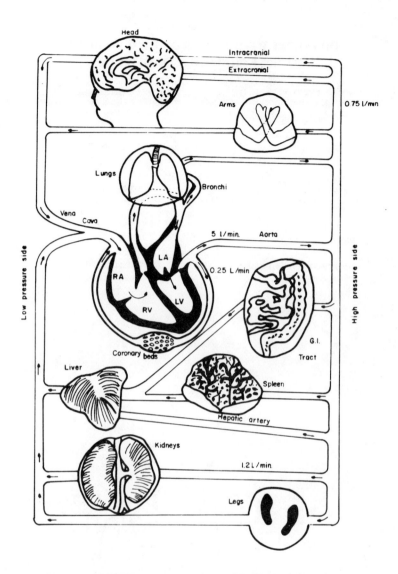

FIGURE 3. Major organs in the circulation.

ventricle into the aorta through the aortic valve. From the aorta, blood is distributed
to all the organs and tissues, where it passes through the capillaries into the venous
system. Through the venous system and the vena cava the blood, rich in CO_2, returns
into the right atrium. From the right atrium, through the tri-cuspid valve the blood
passes to the right ventricle, and from there via the pulmonary circulation into the
lungs. In the lungs, the high CO_2 content of the blood is changed into oxygen and
returns to the left atrium. From there, through the mitral valve, it enters the left ventricle for the cycle to reconvein. Both ventricles can be considered as pumps operating
in series. It is obvious that two pumps working in series must be fully synchronized
and pump the same amount, otherwise the system will either empty itself or fill itself
with fluids. The mechanism responsible for this synchronization is called Starling's
law of the heart, and will be discussed later.

The mechanism of cardiac muscle contraction, known as cardiac mechanics, will
not be described in detail. It should, however, be noted that the muscles surrounding
the atrium are separated from those around the ventricle, but all of them are sur-

Table 5

PHYSICAL PROPERTIES OF HUMAN BLOOD
(UNDER NORMAL CONDITIONS)

Property		Normal Condition
Blood volume		4000—5000 cc
Viscosity[a]	Whole blood:	3.5 centipoise
	Plasma:	1.8—2.5 cp
Blood specific gravity	Male:	1.057
	Female:	1.052
Blood hematocrit	Male:	0.47
	Female:	0.42
Blood PH		7.35—7.40
Blood pressure	Systolic:	120 mmHg
	Diastolic:	80 mmHg
Oxygen content (arterial)		23 cc O_2/100 cc blood
Cardiac output		4500—5000 cc/min
Heart rate		70—75 beats/min

[a]   The viscosity will change with cell pathology and changes in shear rate.

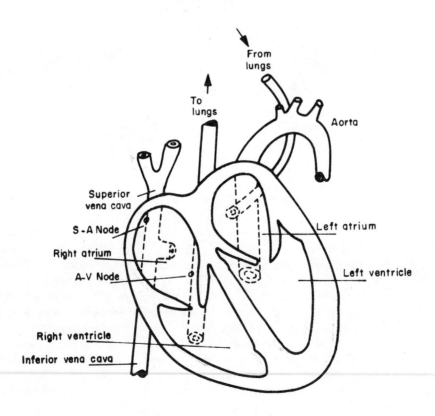

FIGURE 4.   Schematic representation of the heart chambers and flow connections.

rounded by connective tissue. Because of the difference in range of pressure between the right and left atrium, the wall of the left ventricle is much thicker than that of the right ventricle. For additional information on cardiac mechanics the reader is referred to a book with this title by Mirsky et al.[5]

Three parameters are very important for the description of the dynamics of the heart. They are

1. Excitability of the cardiac cells, which determines the action potential and thresholds of excitation.
2. Conductivity, which governs the conduction of the impulse from the cardiac pacemaker to the whole heart.
3. The contractility of the cardiac muscle, which determines the force and pressures generated by the heart.

The signal for the heart to contract comes from the cardiac center located in the medula oblongata (the posterior portion of the brain). It is conducted to the sino arterial node, which is the natural pacemaker of the heart, through the cervical nerve (accelerator). It can also be transmitted through the left or right vagus nerve (depressor) to the atrio-ventricular node. The signal initiates at the sino-atrial node is transferred by conduction to all parts of the heart causing them to contract. The control of heartbeat will be discussed in Section F of this chapter. The contraction of cardiac muscles are raising the pressure inside the heart chambers, this will control the opening and closure of the various valves within the heart, and hence blood flow from one chamber to another as well as blood flow into the systemic and pulmonary circulation.

The supply of blood to the heart itself is carried out by two main coronary arteries that branch off the aorta and supply the left and right side of the heart by further branching. Each branch leads to a terminal artery in charge of very small regions in the heart. The interconnections between the branches are very small in number. As a result any disturbance to blood flow in one of the coronary arteries may lead to an insufficient supply to a certain part of the cardiac muscle leading to necrosis of the area. This in turn leads to deterioration of the muscle in this area and consequently to what is considered, under the general term, heart attack. The blood returns from the cardiac muscle, through the coronary sinus, by the two great middle veins into the right atrium.

An understanding of the hydraulic action of the heart requires an analysis of the mechanical events of the cardiac cycle and the pressures associated with these events during the cycle.

The cardiac cycle is divided into two major parts, systole and diastole, Figure 5. Prior to systole, the atrial pressure exceeds the ventricular pressure by 1—2 mmHg. Hence the mitral valve (the intake valve for the left ventricle) is open. The aortic valve is closed, since aortic pressure is then much higher than ventricular pressure. By activation of the ventricular myocardium the ventricular pressure rises very steeply, for about 0.05 sec, until it reaches the aortic pressure. Immediately after the beginning of the pressure rise the mitral valve snaps shut (producing heart sound I), and the contraction is done with both intake and output valve closed. Hence during this phase the blood volume remains the same and this phase is called isometric contraction. When the ventricular pressure gets to be higher than the aortic pressure, the aortic valve opens and blood ejects from the ventricle into the aorta. This ejection phase is divided into two parts, the first is a rapid ejection where the ventricular volume falls sharply, and the other is a slower ejection. The pressure in the aorta will exceed the ventricular pressure at this phase due to a change from kinetic energy to pressure. After the ejection the myocardium begins to relax and the diastolic phase begins. It begins with a

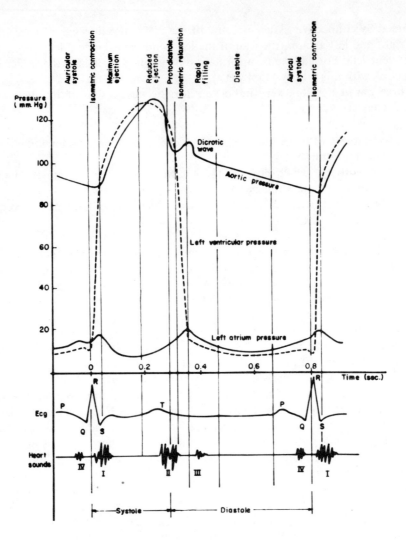

FIGURE 5.   Pressures during the cardiac cycle.

very rapid drop of the ventricular pressure to below aortic level, closing the aortic valve (heart sound II). After this phase, Protodiastole, the pressure continues to drop, with both valves again closed, until it reaches the atrium pressure. During this phase, isometric relaxation, the bulk of blood transferred to the aorta empties to the peripheries and the aortic pressure declines. When the ventricular pressure falls below the atrial pressure the mitral valve opens (heart sound III) and rapid filling of the ventricle takes place, which after that levels off when the atrium contracted, the diastole phase. The most important factor in determining the amount of blood that will flow from the left ventricle into the aorta (stroke volume) is the ventricular filling. The difference between the ventricular volume at the beginning of systole and the end-diastolic volume (EDV) is determined by the energy of contraction of the heart muscle. This will be discussed in Section E of this chapter.

However, many factors effect the ventricular filling. Factors which will increase the ventricular filling are

1.   The central nervous system.

2. Low transthoracic pressure, due to aspiratory action of thorax called also valsalva effect.
3. The diastolic time interval.
4. Slow heart rate.
5. The systolic pressure in the aorta.

Factors that will limit the ventricular filling are (1) the normal resistance of the heart muscle to stretching and (2) the pericardial restrain, which is a pericardial sac (tamponage) that covers the heart and expands and contracts together with the heart.

From the pressure difference between the arterial and venous sides and the average cardiac output the amount of energy delivered by the heart can be calculated, giving a value of 1 W. This is only 15 to 25% of the total energy produced by the heart, since nearly 62% is used for the internal work of contraction of the contractile elements in the cardiac muscle and nearly 23% is required for the maintenance of heart cells. So the heart can be considered a 4-W pump with 20% efficiency.

D. The Pulmonary Circulation

The physiological role of the pulmonary circulation is entirely different from the systemic circulation, and therefore there are marked differences between them.

The pulmonary system carries three different tasks.

1. The main function of the pulmonary system is the exchange of oxygen and CO_2 between the flowing blood and the air in the alveolar space. This gas exchange is done by diffusion. Since it takes a red blood cell only 0.75 to 1 sec to traverse the pulmonary capillaries, or even down to 0.25 to 0.30 during exercise, the contact area must be very large, and the diffusion distance very short. Indeed the surface area is about 100 m², and the diffusion distance less than 10 μm. Hence the system is very sensitive to fluid accumulation on the capillaries inside the alveolar space. If part of the lobes are damaged the internal control will shut down this area and will direct the blood into other lobes.
2. Reservoir. At any time the volume of blood in the pulmonary vessels is about 1 ℓ. Only less than 100 mℓ are in the capillaries. When a certain region requires a temporary increase of blood supply, the additional amount can be taken from the lung.
3. Filtration of the blood. Emboli materials, like thrombus, air bubbles, or fat, that are formed within the systemic circulation are filtered out while passing through the pulmonary circulation. This can be achieved in the lung because not all the lobes in lungs are active all the time.

The difference in physiological role between the pulmonary and systemic circulations is well expressed in the variations in their physical properties, as summarized in Table 6.

The shape of the pressure waves in the pulmonary circulation are similar to those of the systemic circulation, except the amplitude, which is only 1/6 the amplitude in the systemic circulation. During systole, the right atrial pressure will reach a value of 22 mmHg, and in the pulmonary artery the blood pressure will be 22/8 with an average of 13 mmHg. The left atrial diastolic value (7 mmHg) is the pressure at the pulmonary circulation outlet. So a pressure difference of 6 mmHg will transfer through the pulmonary circulation the same amount that requires 100 mmHg in the circulation system. It should be mentioned that this pressure difference remains nearly constant when the amount of blood flow is increased threefold. This is achieved by opening more lobes for blood transport. Some extreme cases where 14.9 ℓ/min were transferred under a pressure difference of 4 mmHg were reported in the literature, see Hickman.[3]

Table 6
THE MAJOR DIFFERENCES BETWEEN SYSTEMIC AND PULMONARY CIRCULATION

Characteristics	Systemic circulation	Pulmonary circulation
Major function	Nutritional requirement	Oxygenation of blood
Type of tissue supplied	Many kinds	One-alveolar membrane
Distance from heart	Varies - mostly long	Very short
Resistance to flow	High	Low
Hydrostatic pressure	High	Low
A-V pressure difference	High	Low
External conditions	Varies greatly	Homogenous-thoracic cage
Surrounding pressure	Interstitial tissue pressure	Subatmospheric
Blood volume	Large	Small
Control	Local	No local control
Pressure regulation at the capillaries	Precapillary sphincter	No precapillary pressure but smooth muscle in arterioles

E. Starling's Law

It is obvious that if the heart can increase its cardiac output up to five times its normal value, there should be a mechanism responsible for control and execution of this process. There are two basic mechanisms of control of the pumping action of the heart: (1) Internal mechanism of control based upon the ventricular filling of the heart (the amount of blood flowing into the heart), and (2) Reflex mechanism of the autonomous nervous system. Starling's law deals with the internal mechanism of control.

The amount of flow transferred to the peripheral system is controlled by the resistance of each region in the periphery. These resistances are connected in parallel, hence, even if the change in a local area of the periphery might be changed drastically the effect on the entire flow is small. This is because the effect on the total resistance is small, and it is the total resistance that determines the total cardiac output. The change in flow resistance is not completely controlled by the capillaries at the peripheral tissues or organs. There might be also changes in the vascular resistance by passive and active mechanisms, as given in Table 7.

The heart must therefore handle any quantity of blood that is determined by all these control mechanisms. The mechanism by which this adjustment is achieved is called Starling's law of the heart.

In simple form the law states that: "The energy of contraction of the ventricular muscle is a function of the length of the muscle fiber". The muscle fibers length at the beginning of contraction are functions of the ventricular filling, and the stroke volume is a function of the energy of contraction. Hence Starling's law can be defined in an alternative way: If the amount of blood flowing into the heart will be higher, the stroke volume will increase by the equivalent value. This means that the heart will respond to a higher input by increasing the output (increased energy) thus keeping material balance. Since the capacity of the heart to store additional fluids is very limited this mechanism should respond in few heart beats (few seconds). Because flow rates at the pulmonary and systemic circulation is equal at all times we can state that a shift of blood quantities from one organ (or tissue region) to another will have the same effect on both atriums and ventricles. A nice example of what would happen if this mechanism did not exist, and one pump will pump a different amount is described by Burton.[1] It is clear that the flow rate at each beat might be slightly different, but on an average, they must be equal.

For example, when inhaling a large quantity of air and holding it, there is an increase of pressure in the thoracic cage, thus decreasing the right ventricular pressure. When

Table 7
FACTORS EFFECTING
VASCULAR RESISTANCE

1. Passive
   a. Distending pressure of vessels
   b. Lung volume
   c. Blood viscosity
   d. Structural changes
2. Active
   a. Local and systemic hypoxia[a]
   b. Local and systemic acidosis[b]
   c. Alkalosis[c]

[a] Hypoxia - Oxygen deficiency at the tissue level.

[b] Acidosis - Acids are absorbed in excess of their elimination, or formed in excess of their neutralization.

[c] Alkalosis - Alkalies are absorbed in excess of their elimination, or formed in excess of their neutralization. Also happens due to prolonged loss of acid from the stomach.

inhaling this air the outflow from the right side of the heart is increased, being higher than that of the left side. This will cause (few beats later) a higher filling of the left ventricle, and, according to Starling's law, a higher outflow.

A simple engineering solution to this problem would have been a shunt between the two systems to transfer excessive amounts from one system to another. The problem with such a shunt is the difficulty of maintaining the pressure within specified limits and relatively fixed. Nevertheless, there is such a shunt through the bronchial artery. And it might be that in a cause of heart failure, when Starling's law does not apply, this shunt takes over the control. This, however, was not proven to be true.

F. Control and Regulation

The summary, in this section, covers very briefly the essential elements of the blood circulation control system. The control center is considered to be composed of three different departments. The measuring apparatus, central interpretation section and command center. The microscopic mechanism of sensing and transmitting the information through the nervous system, is not discussed.

There are various kinds of organs in the human body that must be assured of adequate blood circulation at all times. The amount of fluctuation that each organ can tolerate varies according to its function. The brain, which has the highest priority, must have an almost constant supply of blood at all times. The heart, for example, will tolerate small changes, while the lungs can tolerate great changes in blood supply. Therefore the control of the circulation is achieved by local control at a single organ, or single tissue region, level. Different organs will therefore use different control mechanisms, Figure 6. The apparatus for the flow control can be either the driving pressure or the resistance to flow. But each of them will depend on some other physical properties as seen in Figure 7. The way some of these physical parameters depend on various

1. Metabolic control

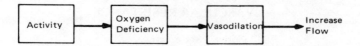

Characteristics of the following organs:
    Brain (this is the only control)
    Heart (very strongly dominates)
    Skeletal muscle

2. Nervous control

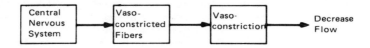

Characteristics of the following organs:
    Skin
    G.I. Tract
    Kidneys
    Skeletal muscle

FIGURE 6.   Control of blood flow to organs.

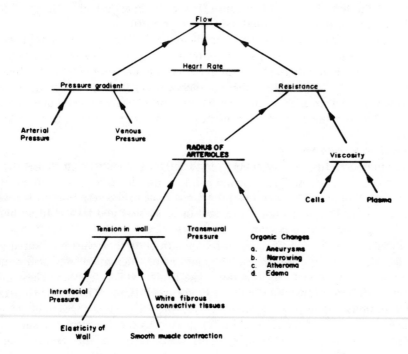

FIGURE 7.   Determination of flow in the systemic circulation.

Table 8
FACTORS THAT DETERMINE HEART RATE

Heart rate accelerated by:

[a] Decreased activity of baroreceptors in the arteries, heart, and pulmonary circulation
[a] Inspiration
[a] Excitement
[a] Anger
[a] Most painful stimuli
[a] Hypoxia
[a] Exercise
[a] Norepinephrine
   Epinepherine
   Thyroxin
   Fever
   Bainbridge effect

Heart rate slowed by:

[b] Increased activity of baroreceptors
[b] Expiration
[b] Fear
[b] Grief
   Stimulation of pain fibers in trigeminal nerve
[a] Increased intracranial pressure

[a] Also produces a rise in blood pressure.
[b] Also produces a fall in blood pressure.

From Ganong, W. F., *Review of Medical Physiology*, Lange, Los Altos, Calif., 1967, 481. With permission.

situations or different agents is summarized in Tables 8, 9, and 10. Factors that determine the viscosity of the blood will be discussed in Chapter 3.

For further discussion the reader is referred to Burton,[1] or for a mathematical description of the control system to Talbot and Gessner.[8]

Appendix 1
POISEUILLE FLOW THROUGH A RIGID CIRCULAR TUBE

Consider a laminar flow of fluid through a rigid cylindrical tube with a circular cross-section. Assume that the tube is very long, so that end effect can be neglected and the flow is fully developed. This will enable the use of a one-dimensional flow. The tube's radius is R, and the fluid density is constant, ϱ. Consider a segment of the tube of length L. In this segment, for any size of concentric cylinder within the tube the momentum balance can be considered. The forces acting on such a cylinder, Figure 8, are the pressures forces on both circular ends (ignore gravity force) and friction at the circumference. These friction forces are the shear stresses, τ. Thus the balance of forces yields:

$$2\pi rL \cdot \tau = (P_1 - P_2)\,\pi r^2 \tag{8}$$

from this relation it follows that

Table 9
FACTORS THAT
DETERMINE THE
RADIUS OF THE
ARTERIOLES

Constriction

Increased adrenergic discharge
Circulating catecholamines (except
  epinephrine in skeletal muscle)
Circulating angiotensin II
Locally released serotonin
Decreased local temperature

Dilatation

Decreased adrenergic discharge
Activation of cholinergic dilators
Histamine
Kinins
"Axon reflex"
Decreased 0_2 tension
Increased CO_2 tension
Decreased pH
Lactic acid, etc.
Increased local temperature

From Ganong, W. F., *Review of
Medical Physiology,* Lange, Los Altos, Calif., 1967, 473. With permission.

$$\tau = \frac{(P_1 - P_2)}{2L} \cdot r \tag{9}$$

This is a relation between shear stresses and pressures. To obtain a relation between pressures and velocity field the relation between shear stress and velocity must be known. An assumption is used here that the relation between the shear stress and the velocity gradient is linear. This relation defines a fluid known as Newtonian fluid. A more detailed definition as well as the use of other nonlinear relation is discussed in Chapter 3.

The ratio between shear stress and velocity gradient, which assumed here to be constant is called dynamic viscosity and is denoted by μ

$$\tau = -\mu \frac{dv}{dr} \tag{10}$$

Inserting this relation into Equation 9 results in the following differential equation:

$$-\mu \frac{dv}{dr} = \frac{P_1 - P_2}{2L} \cdot r \tag{11}$$

Which upon integration, and the use of the no-slip conditions at the wall gives the following solution:

Table 10
FACTORS THAT
DETERMINE TENSION IN
THE SMOOTH MUSCLE IN
THE ARTERIOLES

Tension Increases with:

1. Increasing fiber length
2. Decreasing temperature (cold)
3. Increasing concentration of vasoconstrictive substances such as:
   a. Epinephrine (except in muscle)
   b. Norephinephrine
   c. Angiotensin
   d. Vasopressin
   e. Vasoconstrictor drugs
4. Nervous effects

Tension Decreases with:

1. Decreasing fiber length
2. Increasing temperature (warmth)
3. Increasing concentration of vasodilative substances such as:
   a. Acetylcholine
   b. Epinephrine (only in muscle)
   c. Metabolic (especially CO_2)
   d. Estrogens (in reproduction organs)
   e. Vasodilator drugs
4. Nervous effects

$$V = \frac{P_1 - P_2}{4\mu L} \, R^2 \left[1 - \left(\frac{r}{R} \right)^2 \right] \tag{12}$$

This is called the Poiseuille law or the Hagen-Poiseuille law.
From this equation the following results can be obtained:

1. Maximum flow will occur at the center of the tube and is equal to

$$V_{max} = \frac{P_1 - P_2}{4\mu L} \cdot R^2 \tag{13}$$

2. The average velocity, calculated by integration over the tube's cross section and division by the cross-sectional area, is

$$\overline{V} = \frac{P_1 - P_2}{8\mu L} \, R^2 = \tfrac{1}{2} V_{max} \tag{14}$$

3. The volume flow rate is given by

$$Q = \frac{\P (P_1 - P_2)}{8\mu L} R^4 \tag{15}$$

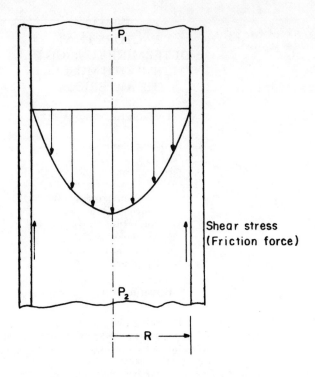

FIGURE 8.   Velocity distribution in flow in circular cylindrical tube.

4.   The velocity profile associated with Poiseuille flow is parabolic. This is true as long as the flow is laminar. It is usually assumed that the flow in a rigid tube is laminar if Reynolds number defined as:

$$R_e = \frac{U \cdot D \cdot \rho}{\mu} = \frac{U \cdot \rho}{\nu} \tag{16}$$

is less than 2000. The value ν is defined as the kinematic viscosity, and is given by:

$$\nu = \frac{\mu}{\rho} \tag{17}$$

REFERENCES

1. Burton, A. C., *Physiology and Biophysics of the Circulation,* Year Book Medical Pub., Chicago, 1965.
2. Ganong, W. F., *Review of Medical Physiology,* Lange, Los Altos, Calif., 1967.
3. Hickman, J. B., A trial septal defect. A study of intracardiac shunts, ventricular outputs, and pulmonary pressure gradient, *Am. Heart J.,* 38, 801, 1949.
4. Middleman, S., *Transport Phenomena in the Cardiovascular System,* Interscience, New York, 1972.
5. Mirsky, I., Ghista, D. N., and Sandler, H., *Cardiac Mechanics: Physiological, Clinical and Mathematical Considerations,* John Wiley & Sons, New York, 1974.
6. Ruch, T. C. and Patton, H. D., *Physiology and Biophysics,* W. B. Saunders, Philadelphia, 1966.
7. Rushmer, R. F., *Cardiovascular Dynamics,* W. B. Saunders, Philadelphia, 1961.
8. Talbot, S. A. and Gessner, U., *System Physiology,* John Wiley & Sons, New York, 1973.

Chapter 3

PROPERTIES OF FLOWING BLOOD

A. Composition of Blood

Blood is a suspension of particles in an aqueous solution of variable constituents. The aqueous solution, called plasma, serves primarily as a transport vehicle for the various cells that occupy 50% of the total volume. The three most important cells in the human blood are the red blood cells (R.B.C. or erythrocytes), the white blood cells (W.B.C. or leukocytes), and the blood platelets. The types of the various cellular cells and their normal range of properties are described in Table 1. Blood constitutes about 8% of the human body weight, so an average man, 70 kg, will have about 5000 mℓ of blood. From this figure the average number of the various cells can be calculated.

The plasma, which occupies 55% of the blood volume consists of 91% water by weight, 3% proteins, and the remainder is acids, glucose, gas, hormones, antibodies, and enzymes. The specific gravity of plasma is 1.03, very close to blood, its viscosity is 1.2 cp and the pH of the plasma is 7.3 to 7.5.

The white blood cells is the name given to various kinds of cells, described in Table 1, which range in size from 7 to 20 μm (in diameter). They play a major role in fighting disease as carriers of antibodies. Because of the relatively low number of white blood cells, compared with the number of red blood cells, their contribution to the circulatory characteristic parameters is minor and usually neglected. This is not true in some pathological cases, when their number increases very sharply.

The platelets, or thrombocytes, are very small in size, but enormous in number. Because of their small size they are usually considered to be rheologically unimportant. However, because of their role in the clotting process they must be considered in discussion on thrombus formation, or when circumstances are such that they form larger aggregates that travel with the blood stream. One of the major factors in determination of the rheological properties of blood is red cell aggregation. This depends to a very large extent on the interaction of platelets and red blood cells. However, it is the properties of the red blood cells that together with blood plasma are responsible for the mechanical and rheological characteristics of blood.

The red blood cell, shown in Figure 1, consists of a very flexible membrane filled with concentrated solution of hemoglobin. The hemoglobin, which has a normal value of 14.4 g/100 mℓ, consists nearly 33% of the cell weight. The viscosity of hemoglobin is 6.0 cp, five times higher than that of blood (1.2 cp). This is a major factor in the deformability of the red blood cell, which is highly significant in the microcirculation, where it passes through blood vessels of the same, or smaller, diameter. The average diameter of the red cell is 8 μm, and it passes not only through the capillaries, (5 μm in diameter), but also through the endothelial wall, which is of the order of 0.5 μm. To do so the red cell is capable of very large extensions and severe deformation.

Because of the major role of the red blood cells in determining the mechanical behavior of blood, it is very important to know the volume concentration of red cells. This volume concentration, called hematocrit, ranges between 42 to 45% in the normal human. A change in hematocrit will change the flow behavior of blood from Newtonian to non-Newtonians, as will be discussed in the following sections. Some important characteristics of human red blood cells are given in Table 2.

If the flow of blood in the smaller vessels is stopped for a short period, the red blood cells will form chains of closely packed cells, called Rouleaux. This can also happen at low shear rates. The length of the Rouleaux chain is a function of shear rate, and the lower the shear stress the longer the chain of particles stacked flat side to flat side. Another important mechanism, as mentioned before, is the clotting mech-

Table 1

NORMAL RANGE OF VALUES FOR THE CELLULAR ELEMENTS CONCENTRATION IN THE HUMAN BLOOD

	Average cell concentration cells/ml	Approximate normal range cells/ml	Characteristic length μm	Percentage of total volume cells %
Total W.B.C.	9000	4000 − 11000	10 Φ	5
Neutrophils	5400	3000 − 6000		
Eosinophils	270	150 − 300		
Basophils	60	0 − 100		
Lymphocytes	2730	1500 − 4000		
Monocytes	540	300 − 600		
Total R.B.C.			1.9×8.0	91
Female	4.8×10^6			
Male	5.4×10^6			
Platelets	3000000	150000 − 40000	3 Φ	4

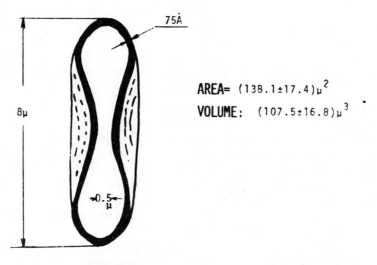

$$AREA = (138.1 \pm 17.4)\mu^2$$
$$VOLUME: (107.5 \pm 16.8)\mu^3$$

FIGURE 1.   Normal shape of red blood cell, with mean dimensions. (From Canham, P. B. and Burton, A. C., *Circ. Res.,* 22, 405, 1968. With permission.)

anism, in which platelets are responsible for the formation of aggregates. These two mechanisms are discussed in more detail in the following sections. It should, however, be mentioned here that the tendency of platelets to form aggregates varies widely in certain diseases.

Many different tests are used in the clinical laboratory to determine various characteristic properties of blood. Besides some tests for blood composition, like blood counts, there are few tests that are related to the rheological properties of blood and plasma. The blood coagulation test, Lee and White method, is performed on venous blood drawn by a syringe. The blood sample is placed in a tube and the time required for coagulation is recorded. It should not be confused with the time it takes a wound to stop bleeding, since in the latter case blood vessel retractility plays a major role. A test that measures this property, the Ivy bleeding test, see Table 1, measures the time it takes a superficial cut 1 mm deep and 10 mm long that lies distal to a 40 mmHg inflated cuff, to stop bleeding. An indirect measure of the Rouleaux formation is the blood sedimentation test. In this test a sample of blood and anticoagulant (5 ml blood

Table 2
NORMAL HEMATOLOGICAL VALUES

Parameter	Symbol	Units	Normal value Male	Normal value Female
Hematocrit	Hct	%	40 − 54	37 − 47
Red blood cells	RBC	Millions/μl	4.6 − 6.2	4 − 5.5
Hemoglobin	Hb	g/100 ml	14 − 18	12 − 16
pH of whole blood	PH		7.35 − 7.45	7.35 − 7.45
Life span		Days	120	120
Mean corpuscular volume	MCV	μm^3	87 ± 7	90 ± 9
Mean corpuscular hemoglobin	MCH	$\mu\mu g$	27 − 31	27 − 31
Mean corpuscular hemoglobin concentration	MCHC	%	32 − 37	32 − 37
Bleeding time (ivy)		min	1 − 7	1 − 7
Coagulation rate (Lee-White)		min	6 − 18	6 − 18
Sedimentation rate				
Wintrobe — under 50		mm/hr	15	20
over 50		mm/hr	20	30

and 2 mg heparin) is placed in a 100 mm long tube (this is the Wintrobe method, but there are a lot of other methods) and after an hour the length of the top layer which is free of particles is measured. Many analytical considerations for the sedimentation tests and their relations to rheological parameters were suggested, for example Ponder, [30,31] and recently Sartory,[35] and Puccine et al.[32]. However, the clinical interpretation is empirical and does not attempt to relate the findings to blood characteristics.

B. Rheological Properties and Viscous Behavior

Before discussing the rheological properties of blood it is necessary to define the various terms that are used to describe the various phenomena associated with viscous behavior.

Viscosity — Many different definitions of this term can be found in the literature. Some are based on microscopic analysis of flow conditions, while others are based on experimentally measurable parameters. A simple definition that can be modified somehow later is: *viscosity is a property of the fluid that determines its resistance for its own motion.* The origin of this resistance can be attributed to adhesion and cohesion forces within the fluid, or more commonly used term with the same meaning, due to friction of fluid layers one against the other.

Analytically this term, μ, defined as the ratio between shear stress and velocity gradient, might depend on various parameters. To start with simple relations, consider a case of one dimensional flow, in the x-y plane, with velocity parallel to the x axis, Figure 2.

The viscosity for this case is given by:

$$\mu = \tau \left/ \frac{du}{dy} \right. \tag{1}$$

Hence, if the velocity gradient is plotted against the shear stress, the tangent to the obtained curve will determine, at each point, the fluid viscosity. Figure 3 gives such a rheogram for different types of flow behavior. The various fluids are defined by their respective rheogram.

Newtonian Fluids — The curve is a straight line that passes through the origin,

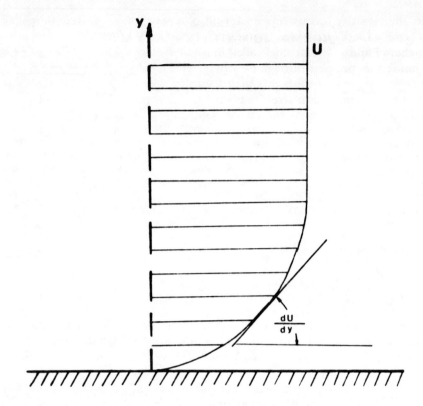

FIGURE 2.   Velocity distribution in one dimensional flow over a flat plate.

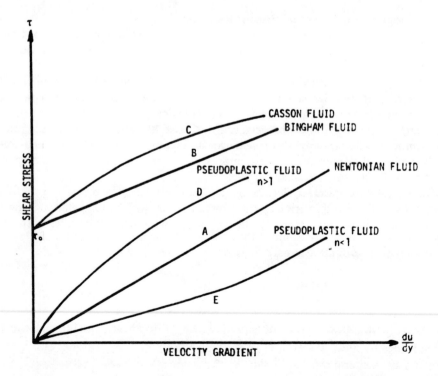

FIGURE 3.   Rheogram for different types of flow behavior, assuming constant pressure and temperature.

hence, the viscosity is constant. It can still be a function of pressure or temperature, but it is not a function of velocity gradient.

Bingham Fluids — Sometimes called Bingham's plastic. The curve is again a straight line, but it does not pass through the origin. This means that to initiate a motion, in a fluid at rest, a shear stress higher than a certain value, τ_o, is needed. The value of τ_o, which is the minimal shear stress that will induce motion is called the yield stress. The relation between shear stress and velocity gradient is given by:

$$\tau = \tau_0 + K \frac{du}{dy} \tag{2}$$

Casson's Fluid — This kind of fluid exhibits the yield stress property of Bingham fluid, but the line is not straight, as shown in the figure. The analytical relation for Casson's fluid is given by:

$$\sqrt{\tau} = \sqrt{\tau_0} + K \sqrt{-\frac{du}{dy}} \tag{3}$$

Casson[9] derived this model for a suspension of particles that form a gel-like aggregate at low shear rate. Equation 3 can be written in the following way

$$\tau = \left(\tau_0 + K^2 \frac{du}{dy}\right) + 2K \sqrt{\tau_0} \sqrt{-\frac{du}{dy}} \tag{4}$$

The first part is a Bingham's fluid behavior, the second part has a power law relation between shear stress and velocity gradient. This is a special case of a more general class of fluids described below.

Pseudoplastic Fluids — Also known as dilitant fluids or Ostwald-de-Waele model. They assume a general power relation, but no yield stress.

$$\tau = K \left(-\frac{du}{dy}\right)^n \tag{5}$$

The family of curves D corresponds to $n < 1$. The E family describes the case where n is larger than 1. The special case $n = 1$ coincides with Newtonian fluid.

In high velocity gradient the deviations of both Bingham and Casson fluids from Newtonian fluids are very small, and can be assumed with very little error that for both fluids

$$\tau = K \left(\frac{du}{dy}\right) @ \frac{du}{dy} \gg 1 \quad \text{or} \quad \tau \gg \tau_0 \tag{6}$$

It is most useful to use in all of these cases the analogy to Newtonian fluids and to define a new quantity, the apparent viscosity

$$\mu_{app} = \tau \bigg/ \frac{du}{dy} \tag{7}$$

It is easier to use this definition in interpretation of experimental results. However, special consideration should be used when studying a fluid that exhibits the yield stress property or pseudoplastic fluid with $n < 1$. In such cases when the velocity gradients tends to zero the apparent viscosity will tends to infinity if this definition is not modified.

Some fluids exhibit rheological properties that depend on the history of flow conditions. This might depend on the history of the velocity gradient or shear rate. These fluids are said to have "memory". Since blood was not found to have these properties and is considered independent of time and history, these kinds of fluids are not considered in more detail.

Usually fluids are divided into only two categories: Newtonian and non-Newtonian. In many published works, even though the fluid is non-Newtonian, the analytical description makes use of the constitutive relations that were developed for Newtonian fluid, with the value of the apparent viscosity at the true viscosity. This is done to overcome mathematical complexity, and introduces an error. However, it enables scientists to reach explicit solutions that could not be achieved otherwise.

C. Viscous Properties of Blood and the Role of Blood Constituents

The value of blood viscosity and its dependence on shear rates have been thoroughly investigated using different measuring techniques, and for various combinations of blood constituents. However, not all the experiments showed the same behavior, and a review of the literature can reveal opposite statements about the viscous behavior of blood components. For example, some researchers claim that plasma behaves as non-Newtonian fluid while others consider plasma a Newtonian fluid. Argument about the validity of blood removed from its natural environment can be found throughout some of the literature.

Some phenomena are agreed by all investigators to take place in blood, yet some investigators call them anomalies of blood behavior.

1. It is well agreed that at low shear rates, the apparent viscosity is markedly increased, and that a certain minimum force, although small, is necessary in order to initiate flow. This suggests an instance of "yield stress", and hence, a Bingham plastic behavior.
2. The viscosity of whole blood decreases with an increase in the rate of shear, this behavior is typical of pseudoplastic fluid.

Hence, the blood can be considered as pseudoplastic with yield stress. As was mentioned in Section B, at very high shear rates the blood behaves as a Newtonian fluid. Because of this it is impossible to have a single analytical expression for describing the rheological properties of blood over the entire range of shear stresses that are found in the human body. Usually some simple expressions for piecemeal fitting over a certain range of shear rate are used for analysis in a specific area where the shear rate is known to be within this limit.

In considering the role of the various constituents of blood it is important to remember that blood viscosity is very sensitive to small variations in its composition and therefore is a very important clinical tool.

Many factors influence blood viscosity and blood flow behavior. Not all the mechanisms by which different parameters affect blood characteristics are fully understood. However, there are a lot of published experimental results on blood flow behavior. Various descriptions of these experiments appear in the literature relating different flow parameters, and using different scaling description. Figure 4 describes one such experiment and the results drawn in three different ways. All of them relate shear rate and shear stress, but neither one of them is convenient for empirical analytical description. Figures 5 and 6 relate shear rate and viscosity, for different values of hematocrit, again using different scales, and again both are not an easy description for analytical interpretation.

It is quite clear from the last two figures that hematocrit plays an important role in

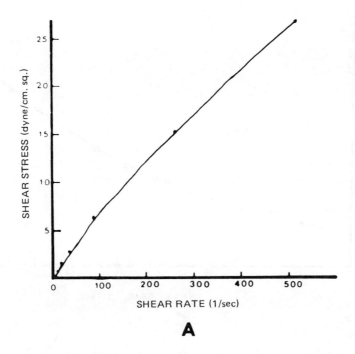

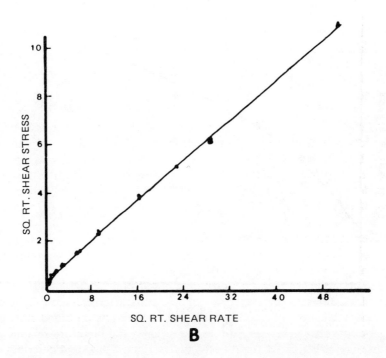

FIGURE 4.   Shear rate vs. shear stress, in various coordinate axes, A through D, for the same experiment, with hematocrit of 46%. (From Rahn, A. W., Tien, C., and Cerny, L. C., *Chemical Engineering in Medicine and Biology*, Hersey, D., Ed., Plenum Press, New York, 1967, 45. With permission.)

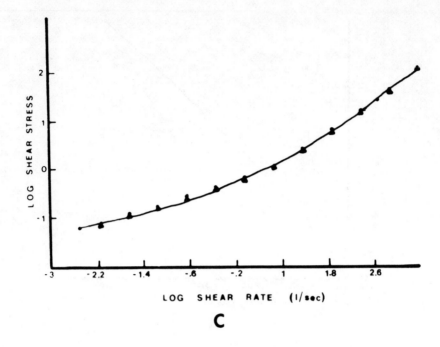

C

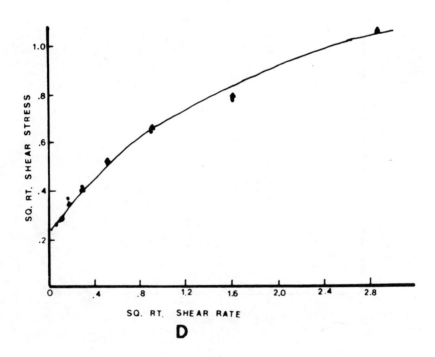

D

FIGURE 4 (continued)

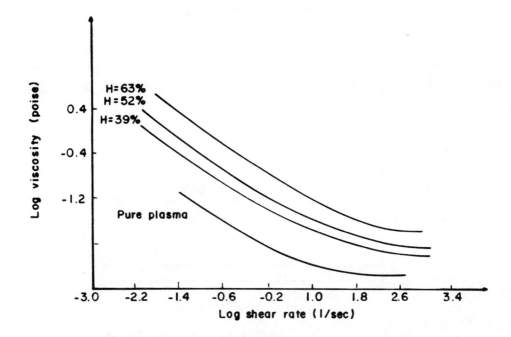

FIGURE 5. Viscosity as a function of shear rate (Log-Log plot) for pure plasma and for different values of hematocrit. (From Rahn, A. W., Tien, C., and Cerny, L. C., *Chemical Engineering in Medicine and Biology,* Hersey, D., Ed., Plenum Press, New York, 1967, 45. With permission.)

determining blood viscosity, and hence, blood flow relations. It is, however, not the only parameter that changes blood viscosity. Not all of these parameters can be discussed separately, since they interact with one another, but considering them by themselves can describe the possible mechanism by which they influence rheological properties of blood.

1. Hematocrit

As was said before, the blood is a suspension of particles in plasma, and the red blood cells are the most important in determining the rheological properties. Hence, in discussing the relation between cell concentration and viscosity the value of hematocrit can be used to approximate the volume concentration of cells. This is undoubtedly introducing a certain error, but since the exact mechanism is not completely known this error is assumed to be very small, and hence, neglected.

The subject of suspension was intensively studied, and thousands of papers published on experimental results and many mathematical models were suggested. However, there does not seem to be any single model that is accepted by all researchers to analytically express the relation between cell concentration and viscosity.

In 1906, Einstein developed an analytical model for the viscosity of suspension of spherical particles in fluid. He assumed low concentration of particles, so that flow around the spheres can be taken as Stokes's flow, which mean no interaction between particles. He obtained the following expression:

$$\mu_s = \mu_p \frac{1}{1 - 2.5c} \simeq \mu_p (1 + 2.5c) \tag{8}$$

where μ_s is the viscosity of suspension, μ_p is the viscosity of plasma, and c the volumic concentration of particles. This relation is accurate up to values of concentration of

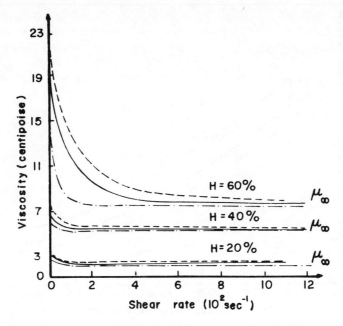

FIGURE 6.   Measured viscosity in a small diameter tube (747 μm
ID). Dashed line (---) indicated apparent viscosity calculated from
Poiseuille's law. Dash-dot lines (-.-.) indicate differential viscosity
which is proportional to the pressure flow curves. Solid lines (– –) are
the generalized viscosity which is proportional to the ratio of applied
stress to shear rate at the wall. (From Haynes, H. R., *Am. J. Physiol.*,
198, 1193, 1960. With permission.)

0.05, where no interaction between particles takes place. In higher concentration, interactions between spheres is important, and should be taken into consideration. This
means that the elasticity of red blood cells, as well as their tendency to aggregate, or
form Rouleaux chain, must be included. This topic is discussed in following sections.

Taylor [42] modified this expression to account for the viscosity of the sphere itself.
This viscosity, denoted by μ_r, is the viscosity of the red cell interior, which is mainly
the viscosity of the hemoglobin. Taylor's expression is:

$$\mu_s = \mu_p \left(1 + 2.5 \frac{\dfrac{\mu_r}{\mu_p} + 0.4}{\dfrac{\mu_r}{\mu_p} + 1} c \right) \qquad (9)$$

This expression also referred to spherical cells and is good for very low concentrations. The idea of particles having other geometry was introduced by Jeffery,[21] who
used a geometrical shape factor, b, as a measure for deviation from a spherical configuration. His analysis leads to the following relation

$$\mu_s = \mu_p \frac{1 + c}{1 - bc} \qquad (10)$$

Other modifications of these relations were suggested by many investigators, as was
summarized by Bayliss.[1] However, all of them relate to dilute suspension with no interactions between particles, and do not fit the description of the in vivo behavior of
blood. All of these relations, and the ones introduced more recently, like Cokelet,[11]

Nubar,[28] and others show good agreement with experimental results in some regions, but a wide deviation in others. Usually the deviations get larger as the concentration increases. This can be due to the inaccuracy of both theoretical model and experimental interpretation of results. Which of these two is more significant cannot be defined very easily, because of a poor reproducibility of the experimental results.

2. Plasma and Serum

The viscosity of plasma depends on the concentration of protein, and generally increases with protein concentration. Although each of the proteins in the plasma has a different effect on the physical properties of plasma and its rheological behavior there are some empirical relations that relate the protein concentration and the plasma viscosity. Bayliss[1] summarizes some of the early models, such as those suggested by the following relation

$$\mu_p = \mu_w \frac{1}{1 - bc} \quad \text{(Hess-Bingham equation)} \qquad (11)$$

where μ_p and μ_w are the viscosities of plasma and water, respectively, c is the concentration of the plasma or serum proteins, and b is a constant.

The relation between blood viscosity and the viscosity of plasma is given by Bayliss as a modified Hatschek equation of Whittaker and Winton:

$$\mu_b = \mu_p \frac{k}{(1 - \phi^{1/3})} \qquad (12)$$

where k is a function of the tube radius and the plasma concentration, ϕ.

The protein found in the higher concentration (50%) in plasma is albumin, but due to its small size its effect on the mechanical properties of plasma is marginal. In some cases a high concentration of albumin is accompanied by a decrease in the concentration of another protein — globulin. This, according to Mayer,[25] causes a decrease in blood viscosity. The average concentration of globulin is 40 to 45%, but in some clinical situations, especially liver disease, it might reach much higher values that may increase the viscosity by a factor of up to 1.5 (Somer[41]). The largest size protein, although the lowest concentration value (5%), that is found in plasma is fibrinogen. The tendency of fibrinogen to form aggregates makes it the most important protein in the determination of the rheological properties. The formation of aggregates, and hence the concentration of fibrinogen, is the dominant factor in producing a yield shear stress in blood, and as such is very important in the determination of flow conditions, especially at low shear rates. Merrill et al.,[26] suggested the following expression for the yield shear stress as a function of fibrinogen concentration

$$\tau_o^{1/2} = 0.36 \left[\frac{B}{1 - C} - 1 \right] \qquad (13)$$

where B is an empirical function of the concentration of fibrinogen in plasma. Another mechanism that involves the fibrinogen is described in the section on added components.

If all the proteins are removed from the plasma, the solution obtained, known as serum, exhibits Newtonian behavior with no apparent yield stress. The viscosity of the serum is lower by about 20% than that of plasma. The most commonly used values for plasma density and viscosity are 1.035 g/mℓ and 0.011 to 0.016 poise, respectively.

3. White Blood Cells

Because the red blood cells outnumber the white (nearly 1000 to 1), the red blood cells will dominate in determining the mechanical coefficients of the blood. However, in clinical cases the production of white blood cells can increase to such a value that the mechanical properties will change. In such cases, the blood exhibits higher values of viscosity and yield stress.

4. Platelets

The fact that platelets are very small in size might lead to the wrong conclusion that their effect on the mechanical properties are minor. However, because of their tendency to clot and form aggregates they can change the whole nature of the flow. Because of the importance of this thrombus formation mechanism it is discussed in a special section.

5. Added Components

Among the components that can be added to whole blood for clinical reasons the most important, in relation to whole blood rheology, are the anticoagulants and dextrans. Both will affect the red cells interactions by changing the electrostatic charge of the erythrocyte membrane. The membrane of the red blood cells is charged by negative ions (Seaman[37]), and surrounding it in the solution there is a layer of counterions that together form a double ionic layer around the membrane. This layer, which extends some tens of angstroms from the cell membrane, plays a major role in forming an electrostatic repelling force to overcome the van der Waals' attraction force between two adjacent cells, and thus to overcome the cells interaction. The presence of proteins in the solution (serum) decrease the attractive van der Waals' force (Kiefer et al.,[23]) thus preventing excessive interaction. However, not all of the added components have the same mechanism, and hence, the same results.

The anticoagulants are added to blood to reduce the degree of interactions and to avoid coagulations. As such they will decrease the amount of yield stress. The overall change in blood rheology, namely the apparent viscosity varies with the type of anticoagulant used. Heparin, for example, decreases the apparent viscosity while citrate will increase the apparent viscosity. Dextrans are added to blood to improve flow conditions, or specifically to increase flow and reduce the rate of shear. Various kinds of dextrans are used, they are divided to those with low molecular weight (smaller than 40,000) which decrease viscosity and decrease the coagulation factor. The other kind, those with molecular weight in excess of 40,000 increase the apparent viscosity and increase the interaction of blood constituents, and hence, the coagulation factor, Brooks and Seaman[2] and Brooks.[3-5]

For further information on the effects and mechanism, of added components the reader is referred to Singh and Coulter[38], Jan and Chein,[20] Brooks[6] and Knox et al.[24] The mechanism of interactions will be discussed in more detail in Chapter 10.

D. Effect of Tube Diameter on Blood Viscosity

In experiments carried out by Fåhraeus and Lindquist[15] using glass tubes of different diameters and constant pressure that was sufficiently high to cause high shear, they discovered that in tubes with diameter smaller than 400 μm there was a substantial drop in "apparent viscosity" and a rise in hematocrit. The apparent viscosity was defined by the slope of Q vs. ΔP curve.

The reduction of apparent viscosity and its dependence on tube diameter, which is called the Fåhraeus - Lindquist effect, is shown in Figure 7. They called their findings an anomalous of blood. Although their observations were correct there is no anomalous in it, and their findings can be explained by two flow mechanisms, (1) the change

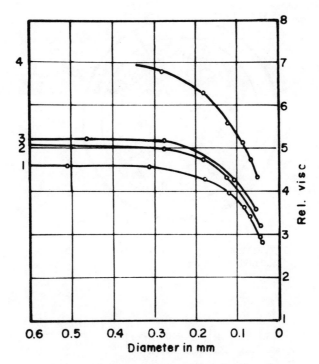

FIGURE 7. The Fåhraeus-Lindquist effect. (From Fåhraeus, R. and Lindquist, T., *Am. J. Physiol.*, 96, 562, 1931. With permission.)

in hematocrit in a tube with a small diameter, and (2) the tendency of the erythrocytes to migrate toward the center of the tube. Both of these mechanisms can be explained analytically.

1. Change in Hematocrit in a Small Diameter Tube

The value used previously as the actual hematocrit of whole blood is an average value, usually obtained by measurement carried out in a sample of blood that was withdrawn from a blood vessel. This, however, is not the real value that exists in flowing blood as will be described by the following argument. Consider two containers connected by a tube of radius R. The containers contain a suspension of particles with a concentration of C_o. Neglect the effect of the length of the connecting tube, and assume that the concentration of particles in the tube is a function of only the distance from the center of the tube, $C = C(r)$, and calculate the average concentration of particles at any cross section of the tube:

$$\bar{C} = \frac{1}{\pi R^2} \int_0^R 2\pi r\, C(r)\, dr = \frac{2}{R^2} \int_0^R C(r) \cdot r dr \qquad (14)$$

At the outlet to the other container the concentration must equal C_o, and hence the ratio of particles arriving at the end and the total flow has to equal the original concentration, namely

$$C_o = \frac{\int_0^R 2\pi r u(r) c(r) dr}{\int_0^R 2\pi r u(r) dr} = \frac{\int_0^R u(r) c(r) \cdot r dr}{\int_0^R u(r) \cdot r dr} \qquad (15)$$

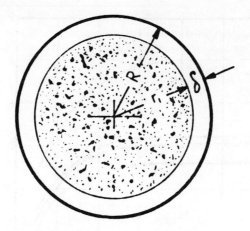

FIGURE 8.   The "free marginal layer" near the wall of the blood vessel.

and hence

$$\frac{\bar{c}}{C_o} = \frac{2}{R^2} \frac{\left[\int_0^R c(r) \cdot r dr\right]\left[\int_0^R u(r) \cdot r \cdot dr\right]}{\int_0^R c(r) \cdot u(r) \cdot r dr} \tag{16}$$

Equation 16 shows that only for C(r) = constant, there will exist $\bar{C} = C_0$. In all other cases the value for the average hematocrit, calculated at any cross section, will be lower than the actual value of hematocrit. It is an obvious result, when taking into consideration the fact that the velocity near the center line is higher than the average velocity, and if the concentration of particles there is also higher, the concentration away from the midline must decrease to maintain the same concentration as in the feeding container. As an example, if the velocity distribution is assumed to be like in Poiseuille's flow and the following concentration distribution is taken for the erythrocytes, the following results are obtained:

linear concentration of particles

$$\frac{\bar{C}}{C_o} = \frac{5}{7}$$

parabolic particles distribution

$$\frac{\bar{C}}{C_o} = \frac{3}{4}$$

all the particles are in an inner layer of radius δ

$$\frac{\bar{C}}{C_o} = \frac{1}{2 - \delta^2/R^2} \tag{17}$$

If the equal concentration on both sides is not enforced, the results are obtained as a function of the diameter of the tube. This is important only in experimental settings. Experimental results on the variation of hematocrit where equal concentration is not enforced are presented by Cokelet.[11]

2. Axial Accumulation of Cells

When introducing a particle of significant size into a fluid stream, two phenomena can be observed. Because of fluid stresses acting on the surface of the particle, it will deform, depending on its elastic properties, it will bend and buckle as well as rotate. This phenomena will be discussed in the next chapter, when discussing the elastic properties of the cell's membrane. In addition to deformation and change in orientation there is an interaction between the particle and the wall of the tube. As a result the particle will migrate in the direction of the axis of the tube due to a net inwardly directed force, usually following a helical trajectory in its migration toward the center line. This usually results in a layer free of particles adjacent to the wall of the tube. This layer, often called the "free marginal layer" or "plasma skimming layer", was observed in blood flowing in arteries and reported by many investigators. Yet there is no complete agreement as to the size of this layer, because of difficulties in measurements.

The migration of particles causes a change in the apparent viscosity of the fluid. Exact analytical treatment of this problem is very complex, since many factors have to be included, such as particle deformability, intra-particle interaction and particle-wall interactions. Most of them were considered separately by various investigators, and some will be discussed in the following chapters. However, a simple analytical treatment can demonstrate how this migration, without consideration of how it is being achieved, affects the apparent viscosity of the fluid.

Assume that due to fluid migration there is a particle-free layer adjacent to the wall. The viscosity of this layer equals the viscosity of plasma, μ_p. The rest of the tube has a distribution of particles and for simplicity it is being considered as a uniform distribution resulting in a uniform viscosity, μ_l. If the free layer is of thickness δ, and the core is of radius $r_l = R-\delta$, the flow in each region, is Newtonian and given by the Poiseuille's solution. The following velocity distribution is obtained

$$U_1 = \frac{1}{4\mu_1} P r^2 + C_1 \qquad o \leq r \leq r_1$$

$$U_2 = \frac{1}{4\mu_p} P(r^2 - R^2) \qquad r_1 \leq r \leq R$$

(18)

where P is the pressure gradient (having a negative value). The continuity of velocities at the interface yields

$$U_1(r = r_1) = \frac{1}{4\mu_1} P r_1^2 + C_1 = U_2(r = r_1) = \frac{1}{4\mu_p} P(r_1^2 - R^2)$$

(19)

$$\therefore c_1 = \frac{P}{4} \left[r_1^2 \left(\frac{1}{\mu_p} - \frac{1}{\mu_1} \right) - \frac{R^2}{\mu_p} \right]$$

The velocity distribution is hence known, and the flow rate can be calculated

$$Q = 2\pi \int_0^{r_1} r u_1 \, dr + 2\pi \int_{r_1}^R r u_2 \, dr = \frac{\pi}{8} P \left[\frac{r_1^4}{\mu_p} - \frac{r_1^4}{\mu_1} - \frac{R^4}{\mu_p} \right]$$

and from this by using the relation

$$Q = -P \frac{\pi R^2}{8\mu_{app}}$$

obtain:

$$\frac{1}{\mu_{app}} = \frac{1}{\mu_p}\left[1 - \left(\frac{r_1}{R}\right)^4\right] + \frac{1}{\mu_1}\left(\frac{r_1}{R}\right)^4 \tag{20}$$

It is clear from this relation that the measured apparent viscosity will yield a value bounded by the two values of μ_p and μ_l. The viscosity μ_l is a function of the particle-free layer δ.

Another approach to the same problem is by considering the tube's cross section as a construction of concentric rings the size of the erythrocyte, and change the integration across the tube by a summation (Haynes[18]),

$$Q = \frac{\P P}{2} \sum_{n=1}^{N} \frac{(n\delta)^3 \cdot \delta}{\mu_n} \tag{21}$$

where $(n\delta)$ replaces r, and δ replaces dr. Assuming that the viscosity can be considered as uniform and taken out of the summation, the apparent viscosity is given by

$$\mu_{app} = \mu\left(1 + \frac{\delta}{R}\right)^{-2} \tag{22}$$

This will always result in a smaller measured viscosity. Although both of these solutions use very crude assumptions and ignore the exact mechanism of fluid migration, they show how such migration can change the measured viscosity, if the Poiseuille solution is considered for the definition of apparent viscosity.

It should be noted that the human body is making use of the fact that near the center line of the tube the concentration of red blood cells, and hence hemoglobin, is higher. In the arterial branches of the kidney and in the main trunk of the uterine artery, there are arterial cushions, Figure 9. These cushions permit "sampling" of blood with a higher value of hematocrit and hence more hemoglobin concentration.[7]

E. The Effect of Slip at the Wall

In deriving the velocity distribution in Poiseuille's flow, Chapter 2, Appendix 1, the boundary conditions that were used were the no-slip condition. However, in the arterial system there are numerous minute branches that carry blood out of the main flow. A simple representation of this arrangement can be made by assuming that the walls of the vessels are made of a porous material. These result in the existence of both radial and longitudinal velocities at the fluid-wall interface. Even if the radial component is very small, and can be neglected, there is still the longitudinal component that must be introduced into the boundary condition. This longitudinal velocity, denoted by S, depends on the wall pores, the shear stress at the wall and the size of particles in the suspension. As a first approximation, Jones'[22] assumption of a constant slip velocity can be considered. This will result in a uniform velocity added to the Poiseuille velocity uniformly across the tube.

$$u = \frac{PR^2}{4\mu}\left(1 - \frac{r^2}{R^2}\right) + S \tag{23}$$

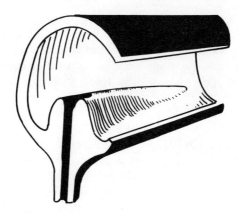

FIGURE 9. Diagrammatic representation of the intraarterial cushions at the origin of a branch of the uterine artery. (From Fourman, J. and Moffat, D. B., *J. Physiol.*, 158, 374, 1961. With permission.)

This results in an additional flow rate, as given by the integration of velocity

$$Q = \int_0^R 2\pi r(u)r \cdot dr = \left(\frac{PR^2}{8\mu} + S\right) \cdot \pi R^2 \qquad (24)$$

The calculated apparent viscosity is obtained by using Poiseuille's flow rate, which is described in the following relation

$$Q = \left(\frac{PR^2}{8\mu} + S\right) \cdot \pi R^2 = \frac{\pi PR^4}{8\mu app} = \bar{u} \cdot \pi R^2 \qquad (25)$$

where $\bar{u}$ is the mean velocity without slip.

The result is always smaller apparent viscosity, given by:

$$\frac{\mu app}{\mu} = \frac{1}{1 + s/\bar{u}} \qquad (26)$$

Jones[22] suggested the simplest possible relation between the slip velocity and the wall shear stress

$$S = k\tau_w \qquad (27)$$

If S is constant the wall shear stress remains the same obtained by Poiseuille's solution

$$\tau_w = \mu \frac{du}{dr}\bigg|_{r=a} = \frac{\mu PR}{2} \qquad (28)$$

and hence

$$\frac{\mu app}{\mu} = \frac{1}{1 + \dfrac{4k\mu^2}{R}} \qquad (29)$$

This oversimplified analysis shows a similar behavior to the Fåhraeus-Lindquist effect, but the mechanism is completely different since they obtained their result in glass tubes with no slip at the wall. This analysis should be used very carefully since it introduces the concept of slip as a continuous slip. In reality a particle moving near the boundaries will be acted upon by a repellent force,[34] causing the particle to move at a slower speed than the continuous (plasma), thus forming a completely different flow condition at the boundaries.

F. Erythrocyte Flexibility and its Effect on Viscosity

In considering the physical properties of an isolated erythrocyte, and predicting from this the gross behavior of the suspension, one must link between the field of microrheology and the field of rheology. This must involve a detailed analysis of the elasto-hydrodynamic characteristics of an isolated erythrocyte and then the effect of cell interactions and interactions with the vessel walls has to be added to produce a gross description. An analytical treatment of this type is too lengthy to be included here, a reference for the material properties of the red blood cell membrane under deformation can be obtained in Skalak et al.,[39] Evans,[14] and Skalak.[40]

The single erythrocyte undergoes shear flow and is subjected to fluid stresses. As a result it will deform. This deformation depends on the shear rate, the cells content, and the elastic properties of the cell membrane.

Since red blood cells lack a nucleus they behave like a fluid drop, and as such the viscosity of the suspension can be described by Equation 9. However, as the red blood cell moves forward, the "red cell membrane can be observed to undergo a tank tread like motion around the red cell content," according to Schmid-Schonbein et al.[36] A more realistic model is Fung's[17] model of a flexible, nonextensible membrane bag, filled incompletely with a viscous, incompressible flow. In high shear rate the deformation of the individual cell is the main factor in the decrease of the relative viscosity. The shear-induced deformation and hence the decrease in relative viscosity all decrease with shear rate. As shear rates get smaller the effect of deformation gets smaller and the cell to cell interactions and cell to wall interactions become the dominate factor.

In considering interactions between cells, the zeta potential of the cell membrane is generating the electrostatic repulsion force between adjacent cells and between individual cells and the walls of the vessels.

It is important to remember that under pathological cases all of these properties will change drastically. For example, sickle cells will undergo deformation in a solid manner.[36] A change in the red cell content results in an increased cell rigidity and higher viscosity. In cases of loss of part of the electric charge, which happens frequently in stored cells, the repulsion force gets lower and this results in higher interaction between cells, increased formation of aggregates, and thus a change in the rheological properties of the blood, as described in the next section.

G. Rheological Aspects of Platelet Thrombosis

Thrombus formation is usually divided into two phenomena. The one occurring in stagnant blood is called a clot. It is a gel, red in appearance, consisting of blood constituents entrapped in a stringy fibrin mesh. It is of importance in sedimentation tests. The other kind of thrombus formation takes place in flowing blood due to collision between particles and interactions between blood particles and the walls of the vessels. This type, which is intensified in cases of contact with an injured tissue or foreign body, produces masses that continue to flow with the blood stream. These masses, called thrombi, consist mainly of platelets, and hence the frequency of collision between platelets is the mechanism that determines the formation of thrombi.

The frequency of collision, and the thrombus size, depends on the local flow conditions, mass transfer by convection, platelet diffusion and diffusion of other chemical species responsible for aggregation. A special attention must be given to special sites in the arterial and venous systems where there are favorable conditions for the formation of thrombi. These places include bents, bifurcations, and sudden changes in lumen diameter.

A detailed analysis of this phenomena is given in Chapter 10. It is, however, appropriate at this stage to determine what is the most probable mechanism of interactions between platelets. It is not clear what are the necessary conditions that are required for two platelets that come in contact to attach and initiate a thrombus. It was mentioned earlier that the electrostatic (zeta) potential of the solution and particles membrane are important, and that some additive will increase the number of interaction. There are also some theories as to the changes that this additive causes. However, there is no unique theory that is accepted by most investigators.

To find out the average number of collisions, Yu and Goldsmith[43] suggested the following calculation. The average value of platelet concentration is 3×10^8 particles/cm^3. In such a case the volume that each particle occupies will be $\frac{1}{3} 10^{-8}$ cm^3, which corresponds to a cube 15 μm $\times$ 15 μm $\times$ 15 μm. Hence, the average distance between the center of two adjacent particles is 30 μm. If the mechanism of platelet motion is assumed to be Brownian translational motion, the diffusion coefficient can be taken as the one calculated by Einstein.[13]

$$D = \frac{KT}{6\pi\mu b} = 1.7 \times 10^{-9} \ cm^2/sec \tag{30}$$

where K is Boltzmann's constant $= 1.38 \ 10^{-16}$ erg/degree; T absolute temperature, (taken as 310K); μ viscosity of plasma (0.012 poise), b equivalent radius of particle ($= 1.1\mu$m).

If the motion is Brownian then this diffusion coefficient is equal to

$$D = \frac{\Delta x^2}{2\Delta t} \tag{31}$$

Where Δx is the random walk at a time unit Δt. Inserting the calculated value for D will result in $\Delta x = 0.6$ μm. This is very small in comparison to the distance between adjacent platelets; and hence to a very small number of collisions. The frequency of two-body collisions between platelets due to Brownian translational diffusion is given by Yu and Goldsmith[43] as:

$$fo = 16 \P nb D = 2.7.10^{-3}/sec \ per \ platelet$$

Hence, if there is no motion, and only diffusion takes place, the number of collisions and the resulting effect of platelet interaction is very small. When sedimentation takes place the distance between particles decreases within the "thick cell area," and interactions will intensify.

For a rough estimation of the average number of collisions in a fluid moving under shear-flow, the presence of red blood cells is ignored, and the blood is considered as a suspension of platelets in plasma. If an average velocity of 15 cm/sec is assumed to take place in a 0.1 cm radius tube, the average velocity gradient is given by:

$$\bar{G} = \frac{2\bar{u}}{R} = 300 \ 1/sec$$

and the average number of collisions is given by:

$$f = \frac{32}{3} \, Gb^3n = 1.3/\text{sec per platelet} \tag{32}$$

Thus under conditions of convective diffusion, the interaction between particles is of fundamental importance. The presence of red blood cells reduces the space available for the platelets. The volume that is left for the platelets to occupy ($\sim$40%) decreases significantly the average distance between adjacent cells, and collision between platelets gets even higher. The effect of motion of the red cells, that results in shear flow in the adjacent fluid, results in higher activity and hence more collisions of the platelets.

Disturbances to the flow stream such as bends, T-joints, bifurcations, and sudden changes in the lumen diameter of the vessel, might result in separation of the streamline, formation of vortex, and backflow. In these regions the velocity gradient might reach a very low (8 to 40 1/sec) or very high (300 to 5000 1/sec) velocity gradient, which might respectively change the number of collisions, as given by Equation 32.

H. Steady State Flow of Fluid With General Constitutive Equation

As was described earlier, the behavior of blood is Newtonian at high shear rate, while at low shear rate the blood exhibits yield stress and non-Newtonian behavior. An analytical description of this fact requires a different description of the relation between shear rate and shear stress in three different regions, see Figure 10. The first region corresponds to low shear rates, and for this region a yield stress and general power low can be considered.

$$\sqrt{\tau} = \sqrt{\tau_0} + \alpha \left(-\frac{du}{dr} \right)^{1/m} \tag{33}$$

α and m are constant. The value of these constants might change for different chemical composition or hematocrit, but they are considered as constant for a given blood sample.

In the third region the flow is Newtonian, and the constitutive equation is given by:

$$\tau = -\beta \frac{du}{dr} \tag{34}$$

The region between the previous two is a transition region. Its boundaries are not definite, and cannot be determined. In an analytical consideration they can be reduced to single point, with shear stress τ_1. This point can be found analytically by any chosen criterion for best fit with experimental results. This will be demonstrated by an example.

Thus the constitutive relation for the whole range of shear stresses can be written as:

$$\frac{du}{dr} = 0 \quad @ \; \tau \leq \tau_0$$

$$\sqrt{\tau} = \sqrt{\tau_0} + \alpha \left(-\frac{du}{dr} \right)^{1/m} \quad @ \; \tau_0 \leq \tau \leq \tau_1 \tag{35}$$

$$\tau = -\beta \left(\frac{du}{dr} \right) \quad @ \; \tau_1 \leq \tau$$

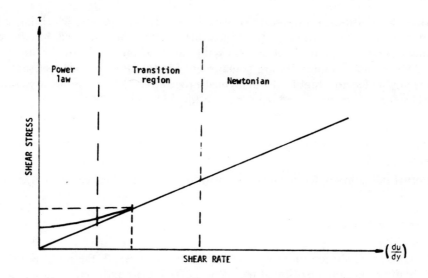

FIGURE 10.   The three regions for the constitutive equation.

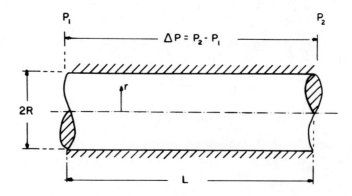

FIGURE 11.   Circular cylindrical tube.

Figure 11 describes a segment of a circular tube of radius R and length L that is subjected to a pressure difference ΔP, resulting in a pressure gradient P, given by:

$$P = -\frac{\Delta P}{L} \tag{36}$$

A balance of the forces acting on a concentric segment of radius r, taken inside the tube results in the following relations

$$-\Delta P \cdot \P r^2 = 2\P rL\tau \tag{37}$$

that results in the following equation for the shear stress

$$\tau = \frac{P}{2} r \tag{38}$$

Since the division to three regions is based on the shear stress, which has a linear relation with the radial distance from the center of the tube, there will be two definite boundaries. However, it is not necessary that all of them will be inside the tube, the cases where these boundaries are actually outside the tube are not real, but can be artificially added to simplify the analytical procedure. The first boundary, R_o, is defined by the yield stress τ_o, and is given according to Equation 38 by:

$$R_o = \frac{2\tau_o}{P} \tag{39}$$

The other boundary is defined by the transition stress τ_l and hence is given by

$$R_1 = \frac{2\tau_1}{P} \tag{40}$$

To make the solution more general it is better to write all the physical properties and geometry in nondimensional parameters. Define a nondimensional parameter D by the following definition

$$D = \sqrt{\frac{PR}{2\tau_o}} = \sqrt{\frac{\tau_w}{\tau_o}} \tag{41}$$

where $\tau_w = PR/2$ is according to Equation 38 the shear stress at the wall. With the introduction of the following nondimensional parameter

$$\Psi = \sqrt{\frac{\tau_1}{\tau_o}} \tag{42}$$

The boundaries are given by the following relation

$$\frac{R_o}{R} = \frac{1}{D^2}$$

$$\frac{R_1}{R} = \frac{\Psi^2}{D^2} \tag{43}$$

Thus, the nondimensional parameters D and Ψ, together with the fluid properties m, α, and β are sufficient for the determination of flow conditions. Three different cases can be defined according to the relative position of the boundaries.

Case 1 — The condition $D < 1$, corresponds to the case where both boundaries R_o and R_l are outside the tube. This means that across the whole tube the shear rate is zero. Because the velocity must vanish at the wall the solution is that of no flow.

Case 2 — The condition $1 < D < \Psi$, corresponds to the case where the first boundary, R_o, is inside the tube and the other boundary, R_1, is outside of the tube. Hence, within the tube there will be only two regions, and the differential equation for the flow is given by:

$$0 < \frac{r}{R} < \frac{1}{D^2} ; \frac{du_1}{dr} = 0 \tag{44}$$

$$\frac{1}{D^2} < \frac{r}{R} < 1 ; \tau = \frac{pr}{2}$$

where τ is given by Equation 33. The solution to the first equation is U_l = constant. The second equation can be combined with Equation 33 to give

$$\sqrt{\frac{pr}{2}} = \sqrt{\tau_0} + \alpha \left(-\frac{du}{dr}\right)^{1/m}$$

or

$$\left(-\frac{du}{dr}\right)^{1/m} = -\frac{\sqrt{\tau_0}}{\alpha} + \left[1 - \sqrt{\frac{pr}{2\tau_0}}\right] = \frac{\sqrt{\tau_0}}{a} \left[D\sqrt{\frac{r}{R}} - 1\right]$$

Raising the last equation to the mth power result is an equation for the shear rate

$$-\frac{du}{dr} = \left(\frac{\tau_0}{\alpha}\right)^m \left[D\sqrt{\frac{r}{R}} - 1\right]^m \tag{45}$$

The last equation can be integrated, with the constant of integration evaluated by the no-slip condition at the wall of the vessel. This results in the following velocity field

$$\left(0 \le \frac{r}{R} \le \frac{1}{D^2}\right) U_1 = \left(\frac{\sqrt{\tau_0}}{\alpha}\right)^m \cdot \frac{2R}{D^2} (D-1)^{m+1} \left[\frac{1 + D(1+m)}{(1+m)(2+m)}\right]$$

$$\left(\frac{1}{D^2} \le \frac{r}{R} \le 1\right) U_2 = \left(\frac{\sqrt{\tau_0}}{\alpha}\right)^m \frac{2R}{D^2} \left\{(D-1)^{m+1} \left[\frac{1 + D(1+m)}{(1+m)(2+m)}\right]\right. \tag{46}$$

$$\left. -\left[D\sqrt{\frac{r}{R}} - 1\right]^{m+1} \left[\frac{1 + D\sqrt{\frac{r}{R}}(1+m)}{(1+m)(2+m)}\right]\right\}$$

An integration of velocities across the tube cross section will yield the volumetric flow rate. This is given by:

$$Q = 2\pi R^3 \left(\frac{\sqrt{\tau_0}}{\alpha}\right)^m \frac{(D-1)^{m+1}}{D^6} \cdot G(D,m) \tag{47}$$

where

$$G(D,m) = \frac{1}{(m+1)(m+2)(m+3)(m+4)(m+5)(m+6)} \star \left\{ D^5(m+1)\right.$$

$$(m+2)(m+3)(m+4)(m+5) + 5D^4(m+1)(m+2)(m+3)$$

$$\tag{48}$$

$$(m+4) + 20D^3(m+1)(m+2)(m+3) + 60D^2(m+1)(m+2)$$

$$\left. + 120D(m+1) + 120\right\}$$

As an example, consider the case m = 2, which corresponds to Casson's fluid model. In this case the velocities and flow rates are given by:

$$\left(0 \le \frac{r}{R} \le \frac{1}{D^2}\right) \quad U_1 = \frac{\tau_0}{\alpha^2} \cdot \frac{2R}{D^2} \cdot (D-1)^3 \frac{1+3D}{12}$$

$$\left(\frac{1}{D^2} \le \frac{r}{R} \le 1\right) \quad U_2 = \frac{\tau_0}{\alpha^2} \cdot \frac{2R}{D^2} \left\{ (D-1)^3 \frac{1+3D}{12} - \left(D\sqrt{\frac{r}{R}}-1\right)^3 \frac{1+3D\sqrt{\frac{r}{R}}}{12} \right\} \tag{49}$$

$$Q = 2\pi R^3 \frac{\tau_0}{\alpha^2} \frac{21D^8 - 48D^7 + 28D^6 - 1}{168D^6}$$

This result for Casson's fluid was first presented by Oka,[29] but is presented here in a different form that permits an easier identification of the specific flow cases.

Case 3 — In this case all the boundaries are within the tube. This corresponds to

$$D > \Psi = \sqrt{\frac{\tau_0}{\tau_1}}$$

Thus there are three different regions, and the differential equations that describe the flow conditions are

$$0 \le \frac{r}{R} \le \frac{1}{D^2} \; ; \; \frac{du_1}{dr} = 0$$

$$\frac{1}{D^2} \le \frac{r}{R} \le \frac{\Psi^2}{D^2} ; \left(-\frac{du_2}{dr}\right) = \left(\frac{\tau_0}{\alpha}\right)^m \left[D\sqrt{\frac{r}{R}} - 1 \right]^m \tag{50}$$

$$\frac{\Psi^2}{D^2} \le \frac{r}{R} \le 1 \; ; \; \frac{du_3}{dr} = -\frac{Pr}{2\beta}$$

A simple integration of these equations results in the following solution.

$$U_1 = K_1$$

$$U_2 = \left(\frac{\sqrt{\tau_0}}{\alpha}\right)^m \frac{2R}{D^2} \left\{ \frac{\left[D\sqrt{\frac{r}{R}} - 1 \right]^{2+m}}{2+m} + \frac{\left[D\sqrt{\frac{r}{R}} - 1 \right]^{1+m}}{1+m} \right\} + K_2 \tag{51}$$

$$U_3 = -\frac{Pr^2}{4\beta} + K_3$$

The constants can be determined from the boundary condition and the condition of continuity

$$U_3 = 0 \quad @ \quad r = R$$

$$U_2 = U_3 \quad @ \quad r = R_1 \tag{52}$$

$$U_1 = U_2 \quad @ \quad r = R_0$$

And the solution is given by the following equations

$$\left(0 \le \frac{r}{R} \le 1/D^2\right) \ U_1 \ = \ \frac{PR^2}{4\beta}\left[1 - \frac{\Psi^4}{D^4}\right] + \left(\frac{\sqrt{\tau_0}}{\alpha}\right)^m \frac{2R}{D^2}\left\{\frac{[\Psi - 1]^{2+m}}{2+m} + \frac{[\Psi - 1]^{1+m}}{1+m}\right\}$$

$$\left(\frac{1}{D^2} \le \frac{r}{R} \le \frac{\Psi^2}{D^2}\right) \ U_2 \ = \ \frac{PR^2}{4\beta}\left[1 - \frac{\Psi^4}{D^4}\right] + \left(\frac{\sqrt{\tau_0}}{\alpha}\right)^m \frac{2R}{D^2}\left\{\frac{[\Psi - 1]^{2+m}}{2+m} + \frac{[\Psi - 1]^{1+m}}{2+m}\right\} \quad (53)$$

$$- \left(\frac{\sqrt{\tau_0}}{\alpha}\right)^m \frac{2R}{D^2}\left\{\frac{\left[D\sqrt{\frac{r}{R}} - 1\right]^{2+m}}{2+m} + \frac{\left[D\sqrt{\frac{r}{R}} - 1\right]^{1+m}}{1+m}\right\}$$

$$\left(\frac{\Psi^2}{D^2} \le \frac{r}{R} \le 1\right) \qquad\qquad U_3 \ = \ \frac{PR^2}{4\beta}\left[1 - \left(\frac{r}{R}\right)^2\right]$$

Again the volumetric flow rate can be obtained from direct integration of these equations.

$$Q = 2\pi \int_0^{R/D^2} U_1\, r dr + 2\pi \int_{R/D^2}^{R\Psi^2/D^2} U_2\, r dr + 2\pi \int_{R\Psi^2/D^2}^{R} U_3\, r dr \qquad (54)$$

The following expression is obtained, after integration

$$Q = \frac{2\pi PR^4}{16\beta D^8}(D^8 - \Psi^8) + 2\pi \left(\frac{\sqrt{\tau_0}}{\alpha}\right)^m \frac{R^3}{D^6}(\Psi - 1)^{1+m}\, G(\Psi, m) \qquad (55)$$

where $G(\Psi, m)$ is given by Equation 48.

In the limiting case, where Ψ approaches D, this solution will coincide with the solution of Case 2, thus providing continuity.

As will be seen in some examples to follow this discussion the values of τ_0, α and m vary with hematocrit, chemical composition and disease. However, Equation 47 can be written in the following form

$$Q' = \frac{Q}{2\pi R^3 \left(\frac{\sqrt{\tau_0}}{\alpha}\right)^m} = f(D, m) \qquad (56)$$

This is a general form that permits us to draw Q' vs D for different values of m. This is shown in Figure 12. However, this cannot be done for the third case, since we have two additional fluid parameters β and Ψ.

As was indicated earlier the general constitutive equation is reduced in the special case of m = 2 to Casson's equation. If at the same time the yield stress, τ_0, is approaching the value of zero, these solutions will approach the Poiseuille case with α^2 as the fluid viscosity.

Example 1

Merrill and Pelletier[27] suggested the adoption of Casson's equation to describe blood flow. As an example, consider from their results (sample 149), for which they suggested the following relations

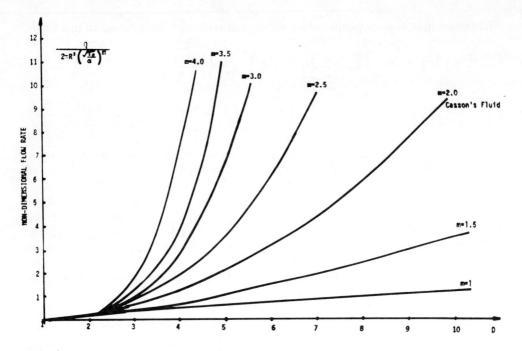

FIGURE 12.   Nondimensional flow rate, for fluids with various values of m, as a function of the nondimensionalized parameter D.

$$\text{At low shear rates:} \quad \sqrt{\tau} = 0.20 + 0.1738 \sqrt{\frac{-du}{dr}}$$

$$\text{At high shear rates:} \quad \sqrt{\tau} = 0.18 \sqrt{\frac{-du}{dr}}$$

$$(57)$$

These relations were obtained experimentally for a sample with 40% hematocrit, and fibrinogen concentration of 0.27. This corresponds to the following assigned parameters

$$\tau_0 = 0.04 \ \text{dyn/cm}^2$$

$$\beta = 0.0324 \ \text{dyn} \cdot \text{sec/cm}^3$$

$$\alpha = 0.01738 \ (\text{dyn} \cdot \text{sec/cm}^2)^{1/2}$$

$$m = 2$$

Equation 49 describes the velocity distribution for Case 2, where only one boundary lies within the tube. The velocity field for these parameters, under Case 3, where both boundaries are within the tube, is given by the following relations

$$\left(0 \le \frac{r}{R} \le 1/D^2\right) \ U_1 = \frac{\tau_0}{\alpha^2} \cdot \frac{2R}{D^2} (\Psi - 1)^3 \frac{1 + 3\Psi}{12} + \frac{PR^2}{4\beta} \left(1 - \frac{\Psi^4}{D^4}\right)$$

$$\left(1/D^2 \le \frac{r}{R} \le \Psi^2/D^2\right) \ U_2 = \frac{\tau_0}{\alpha^2} \cdot \frac{2R}{D^2} \left\{ (\Psi - 1)^3 \frac{1 + 3\Psi}{12} - \left(D\sqrt{\frac{r}{R}} - 1\right)^3 \frac{1 + 3D\sqrt{\frac{r}{R}}}{12} \right.$$

$$\left. + \frac{PR^2}{4\beta} \left(1 - \frac{\Psi^4}{D^4}\right) \right\}$$

$$(58)$$

$$\left(\Psi^2/D^2 \le \frac{r}{R} \le 1\right) \qquad U_3 = \frac{PR^2}{4\beta} \left[1 - \frac{r^2}{R^2}\right]$$

The transition region, as defined by Merrill and Pelletier[27] can be reduced to a single point by taking the point in the center of transition region, which, given $\tau_o = 1.41$ dyn/cm^2, gives

$$\Psi = \sqrt{\frac{\tau_1}{\tau_o}} = 5.94$$

These values can be inserted into the equations, and flow conditions can be calculated. The velocity distribution for this case is given in Figures 13 and 14. It can be seen that only at low values of the nondimensional parameters D there is a measurable plug flow near the center of the tube. Figures 15 and 16 describe the flow rates for different values of D, and compared with the flow that would exist if the same pressure gradient and tube diameter are considered with a Poiseuille's flow of fluid with no yield stress and viscosity equal to $\beta = 0.0324$ poise. In the calculation of the Poiseuille's flow rates the value of τ_o is considered as a constant, and has no physical meaning. It is shown that there is a difference at low value of D, where the actual flow rate of this sample is smaller than that predicted by Poiseuille's flow. This explains why the apparent viscosity, Figure 17, based on Poiseuille's profile has this shape, that was found by many investigators.

Example 2

The example of Merrill and Pelletier[27] confirmed the value of m = 2. However, not all the published experimental results agree with this value. Consider the experimental findings of Rahn et al.[33] The case considered is with hematocrit value of 46%. The best fit for their experimental curve, based on the least square method, shown in Figure 18, yields the following results

for low shear rates: $\sqrt{\tau} = 0.80 + 0.46252 \left(-\dfrac{du}{dr}\right)^{0.66287}$

(59)

and for high shear rates: $\sqrt{\tau} = -0.2358 \sqrt{-\dfrac{du}{dr}}$

Figure 18 shows also the transition region, and the method of reducing this region to a single point. This gives the following values

$$\tau_o = 0.04 \quad \text{dyn/cm}^2$$

$$\sqrt{\tau_1} = 2.50 \quad (\text{dyn/cm}^2)^{1/2}$$

$$\alpha = 0.462525 \, (\text{dyn} \cdot \text{sec/cm}^2)^{1/2}$$

$$\beta = 0.05464 \quad \text{dyn} \cdot \text{sec/cm}^2$$

$$m = 3.02$$

The velocity distribution for this case is described in Figure 19, where the boundary between Case 2 and Case 3, takes place at D = Ψ, given by τ_1 and τ_o, and equals 12.50. The volumetric flow rate is described in Figure 20.

The apparent viscosity, Figure 21, is described as a function of the nondimensional parameter D. When either P is held constant while the radius is decreased, or R is held constant and the pressure gradient P is decreased, the apparent viscosity will reach very high values.

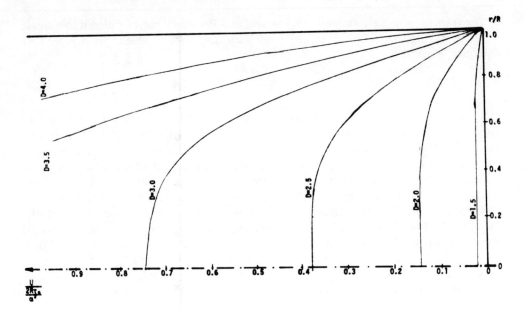

FIGURE 13.   Velocity distribution for a fluid with properties calculated. (From Merrill, E. W. and Pelletier, G. A., *J. Appl. Physiol.*, 33, 178, 1967. With permission.)

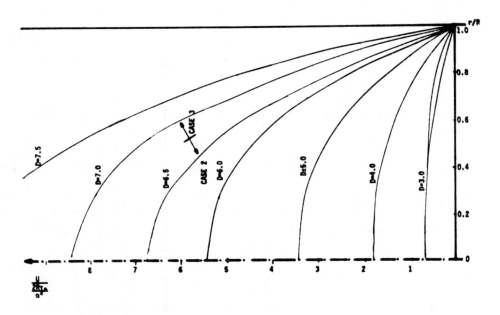

FIGURE 14.   Velocity distribution for a fluid with properties calculated. (From Merrill, E. W. and Pelletier, G. A., *J. Appl. Physiol.*, 33, 178, 1967. With permission.)

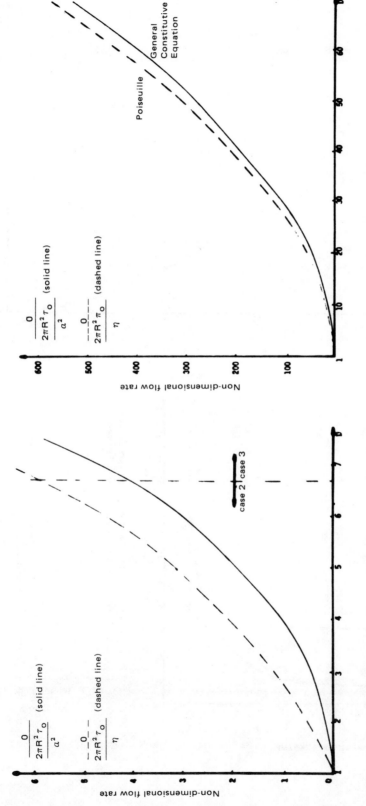

FIGURE 16. The variation of volume flow rate as a function of D, for the general constitutive equation (solid line) and parameters defined from the work of Merrill and Pelletier,[27] and for Poiseuille's flow under the same pressure gradient for the same tube diameter. (In this case τ_o is a constant without any physical meaning, it is introduced in order to use the nondimensional parameter D as variable.)

FIGURE 15. The variation of volume flow rate as a function of D, for the general constitutive equation (solid line) and parameters defined from the work of Merrill and Pelletier,[27] and for Poiseuille's flow under the same pressure gradient for the same tube diameter. (In this case τ_o is a constant without any physical meaning, it is introduced in order to use the nondimensional parameter D as variable.)

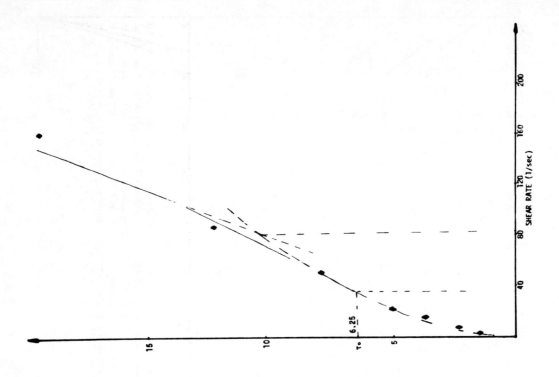

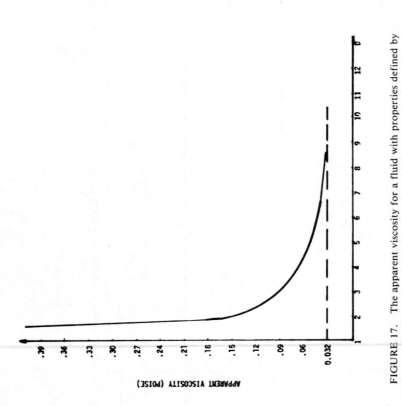

FIGURE 17.   The apparent viscosity for a fluid with properties defined by the work of Merrill and Pelletier,[27] computed with a Poiseuille profile assumption.

FIGURE 18.   The three regions for the general constitutive equation, for best fit to the results of Rahn, Tien and Cerny.[33]

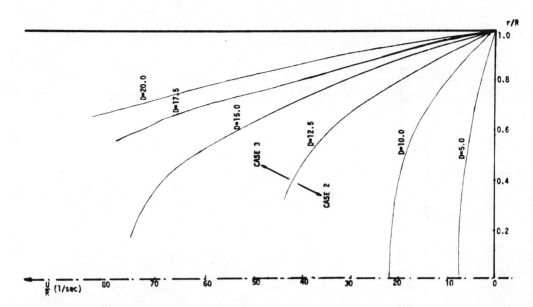

FIGURE 19. The variation of velocity (divided by tube radius) along the cross section of the tube as a function of the nondimensionalized parameter D. The fluid is obeying the general constitutive equation and the parameters calculated from Rahn, Tien, and Cerny.[33]

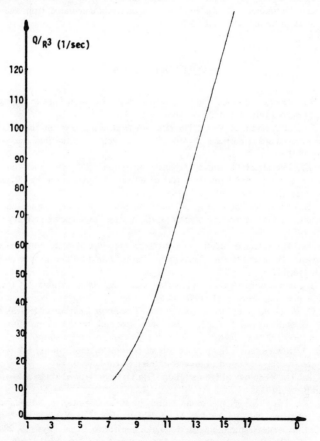

FIGURE 20. Volumetric flow rate (divided by the third power of the tube radius) as a function of the nondimensionalized parameter D, for a fluid with parameters calculated from the work of Rahn, Tien, and Cerny.[33]

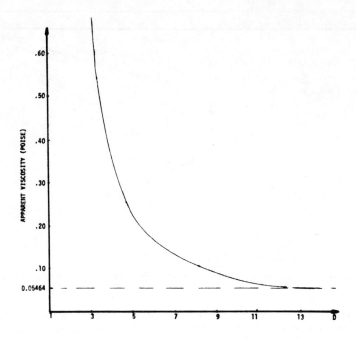

FIGURE 21.   Apparent viscosity as a function of the nondimensionalized parameter D, for fluid with parameters calculated from the
work of Rahn, Tien, and Cerny.[33]

REFERENCES

1. **Bayliss, L. E.**, Rheology of blood and lymph, in *Deformation and Flow in Biological System*, Frey-Wissling, A., Ed., North Holland, Amsterdam, 1952, 354.
2. **Brooks, D. E. and Seaman, G. V. F.**, The effect of neutral polymers on the electrokinetic potential of cells and other charged particles. I. Models for the zeta potential increase, *J. Colloid Interface Sci.*, 43, 670, 1973.
3. **Brooks, D. E.**, The effect of neutral polymers on the electrokinetic potential of cells and other charged particles. II. A model for the effect of adsorbed polymer on the diffuse double layer, *J. Colloid Interface Sci.*, 43, 687, 1973.
4. **Brooks, D. E.**, The effect of neutral polymers on the electrokinetic potential of cells and other charged particles. III. Experimental studies on the dextran/erythrocyte system, *J. Colloid Interface Sci.*, 43, 700, 1973.
5. **Brooks, D. E.**, The effect of neutral polymers on the electrokinetic potential of cells and other charged particles. IV. Electrostatic effects in dextran-mediated cellular interactions, *J. Colloid Interface Sci.*, 43, 714, 1973.
6. **Brooks, D. E.**, Red cell interactions in low flow states, in *Microcirculation,* Grayson, J. and Zingg, W., Eds., Plenum Press, New York, 1976, 33-52.
7. **Burton, A. C.**, *Physiology and Biophysics of the Circulation,* Yearbook Medical, Chicago, 1965, 54.
8. **Canham, P. B. and Burton, A. C.**, Distribution of size and shape in populations of normal human red cells, *Circ. Res.*, 22, 405, 1968.
9. **Casson, N.**, A flow equation for pigment-oil suspension of the printing ink type, in *Rheology of Disperse Systems,* Mill, C. C., Ed., Pergamon Press, Oxford, 1959.
10. **Cokelet, G. R.**, The Rheology of Human Blood, Ph.D. Dissertation, Massachusetts Institute of Technology, Cambridge, 1963.
11. **Cokelet, G. R.**, The rheology of human blood, in *Biomechanics, Its Foundation and Objectives,* Fung, Y. C., Perrone, N., and Anliker, M., Eds., Prentice-Hall, Englewood Cliffs, N.J., 1972, 63.
12. **Einstein, A.**, Eine Neue Bestimmung det Molekuldimensronen, *Ann. Phys.*, 19, 289, 1906.
13. **Einstein, A.**, *The Rheology of the Brownian Movement,* Dover, New York, 1959.
14. **Evans, E. A.**, A new material concept for the red cell membrane, *Biophys. J.*, 13, 926, 1973.
15. **Fåhraeus, R. and Lindquist, T.**, The viscosity of the blood in narrow capillary tubes, *Am. J. Physiol.*, 96, 562, 1931.

16. Fourman, J. and Moffat, D. B., The effect of intraarterial cushions on plasma skimming in small arteries, *J. Physiol.*, 158, 374, 1961.
17. Fung, Y. C., Theoretical consideration of the elasticity of the red cells and small blood vessels, *Fed. Proc. Fed. Am. Soc. Exp. Biol.*, 25, 1761, 1966.
18. Haynes, H. R., Physical basis of the dependence of blood viscosity on tube radius, *Am. J. Physiol.*, 198, 1193, 1960.
19. Haynes, R. H., The rheology of blood, *Trans. Soc. Rheol.*, 5, 85, 1961.
20. Jan, K. M. and Chein, S., Influence of the ionic composition of fluid medium on red cell aggregation, *J. Physiol.*, 61, 655, 1973.
21. Jeffery, G. B., The motion of ellipsodial particles immersed in a viscous fluid, *Proc. R. Soc. (London) Ser. A*, 102, 161, 1922.
22. Jones, A. L., On the flow of blood in tube, *Biorheology*, 3, 183, 1966.
23. Kiefer, J. E., Paroegian, V. A., and Weiss, G. H., Model for the van der Waals attraction between spherical particles with non-uniform adsorbed polymer, *J. Colloid Interface Sci.*, 51, 543, 1975.
24. Knox, R. J., Nordt, F. J., Seaman, G. V. F., and Brooks, D. E., Rheology of erythrocyte suspensions: dextran-mediated aggregation of deformable and non-deformable erythrocytes, *Biorheology*, 14, 75, 1977.
25. Mayer, G. A., Relation of the viscosity of plasma and whole blood, *Am. J. Clin. Pathol.*, 45, 273, 1966.
26. Merrill, W. W., Margetts, W. G., Cokelet, G. R., and Gilliland, E. R., The casson equation and rheology of blood near zero shear, in *Symp. Biorheology*, Copley, A. L., Ed., Interscience, New York, 1965, 135.
27. Merrill, E. W. and Pelletier, G. A., Viscosity of human blood: transition from Newtonian to non-Newtonian, *J. Appl. Physiol.*, 33, 178, 1967.
28. Nubar, Y., The laminar flow of a composite fluid: an approach to the rheology of blood, *Ann. N.Y. Acad. Sci.*, 136, 33, 1966.
29. Oka, S., Theoretical considerations on the flow of blood through a capillary, in *Symp. Biorheology*, Copley, A. C., Ed., Interscience, New York, 1965, 89-102.
30. Ponder, E. J., On sedimentation and rouleaux formation. I, *Q. J. Exp. Physiol.*, 15, 235, 1925.
31. Ponder, E. J., On sedimentation and rouleaux formation. II, *Q. J. Exp. Physiol.*, 17, 179, 1926.
32. Puccini, C., Stasiw, D. M., and Cerny, L. C., The erythrocyte sedimentation curve: a semi-empirical approach, *Biorheology*, 4, 43, 1977.
33. Rahn, A. W., Tien, C., and Cerny, L. C., Flow properties of blood under low shear rate, in *Chemical Engineering in Medicine and Biology*, Hersey, D., Ed., Plenum Press, New York, 1967, 45.
34. Saffman, P. G., On the motion of small spheriodal particles in a viscous liquid, *J. Fluid Mech.*, 1, 540, 1956.
35. Sartory, W. K., Three component analysis of blood sedimentation by the method of characteristics, *Math. Biosci.*, 33, 145, 1977.
36. Schmid-Schumbein, H., Wells, R., and Goldstone, J., Model experiments in red cell rheology: the mannilian red cell as a fluid drop, in *Theoretical and Clinical Rheology*, Hartret, H. H. and Copley, A., Eds., Springer-Verlag, Basel, 1969, 233.
37. Seaman, G. V. F., Electrokinetic behavior of red cells, in *The Red Blood Cell*, Vol. 2, 2nd ed., Surgenor, R., Ed., Academic Press, New York, 1975, 1135.
38. Singh, M. and Coulter, A., Rheology of blood, effect of dilution with various dextrans, *Microvasc. Res.*, 5, 123, 1973.
39. Skalak, R., Tozeren, A., Zarda, P. R., and Chien, S., Strain energy function of red blood cell membranes, *Biophys. J.*, 13, 245, 1973.
40. Skalak, R., Rheology of red blood cell membrane, in *Microcirculation, Blood-Vessel Interactions Systems in Special Tissues*, Grayson, J. and Zingg, W., Eds., Plenum Press, New York, 1976, 53.
41. Somer, T., The viscosity of blood, plasma and serum in dys and paraproteinemias, *Acta Med. Scand.*, 180, Suppl. 456, 1966.
42. Taylor, G. I., The viscosity of a fluid containing small drops of another fluid, *Proc. Roy. Soc. (London), Sec. A.*, 138, 41, 1932.
43. Yu, S. K. and Goldsmith, H. L., Some rheological aspects of platelet thrombosis, in *Platelets, Drugs, and Thrombosis*, Symp. Hamilton, S. Karger, Basel, 1972, 78.

Chapter 4

STRUCTURE AND PHYSIOLOGY OF BLOOD VESSELS

A. Structure and Dimensions of the Arterial Tree

The arterial tree comprises of vessels of various length and diameter that successively branch into smaller vessels. They originate from the aorta and branch until they reach a mesh of very small caliber vessels, the capillaries. The arterial tree is shown in Figure 1. After passing through the capillary bed the vessels combine together to larger and larger vessels to form the venous system, shown in Figure 2. The reduction in diameter, on the arterial side, is achieved not only by branching, but also by a gradual change of diameter, known as tapering of the arteries.

The blood leaves the heart through the aorta, which is firmly attached to the cardiac skeleton at the root of the aorta. It is the largest artery in the body, and averages 3 cm in diameter at the ventricular outlet. The aorta extends upward from the aortic valve, and then descends toward the bifurcation. Along this path the diameter slowly decreases and reaches an average of 1.75 cm at the bifurcation. This section of the aorta is divided into three segments:

1. The ascending aorta, average length 5 cm, which lies between the pulmonary artery and the superior vena cava. Near the origin of the ascending aorta there are only two branches, the right and left coronary arteries, which supply the cardiac muscle with blood.

2. The aortic arch, where the aorta bends to the left and arches backward to about 2.5 cm below the upper border of the sternum. Three branches exit from the top of the arch: the brachiocephalic, the left common carotid, and the left subclavian arteries. The average length of this segment is similar to this of ascending aorta, namely 5 cm.

3. The descending aorta which consists of the descending thoracic aorta, about 20 cm long. The thoracic aorta branches into two major arteries the parietal branches that carry blood to the body wall and the visceral branches that supply blood to organs within the body cavity, and then continue to become the descending abdominal aorta. This segment also branches into parietal and visceral branches and terminates in front of the fourth lumbar vertebra by dividing into the common iliac arteries.

All of these branches are of a relatively large diameter, and because of this the reduction in cross section must be also large. And indeed the aorta has the largest geometrical tapering of all the arteries. These major branches continue to branch further, and hence to further reduce in diameter until they reach the capillary bed. When a specific internal organ, or arterial segment, is to be considered, the average dimensions should be studied very carefully. This can be obtained from various textbooks on human anatomy. Another feature of the arterial tree that has to be considered when analyzing a specific segment, is the existence of direct routes from the arterial to the venous sides. These shortcuts, known as arteriovenous shunts, is of utmost importance and will be considered in depth later.

B. The Structure and Composition of the Blood Vessel Wall

Classification of arteries is usually done by their size, however, another classification that is very frequently used, is by structure. The larger arteries leading from the heart and the first few branches are known as the elastic arteries, because of the large amount of elastin in them. As the distance from the heart increases, the amount of muscle

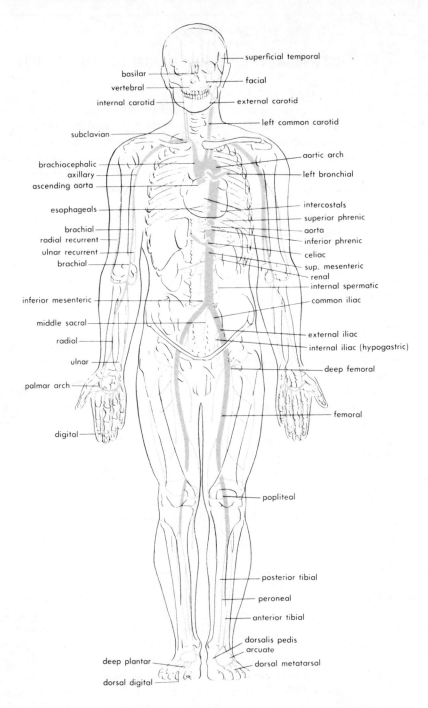

FIGURE 1.   Diagram of the arterial system. (From Crouch, J. E., *Functional Human Anatomy*, 3rd ed., Lea & Febiger, Philadelphia 1978, 432. With permission.)

cells, that lies in rings around the lumen of the artery increases, and the arterial structure transforms to what is known as muscular arteries. This classification is too simple since the two kinds do not differ only by the relative amount of muscle cells or elastin. Five components comprise the vessel wall, and the ratio between them varies according

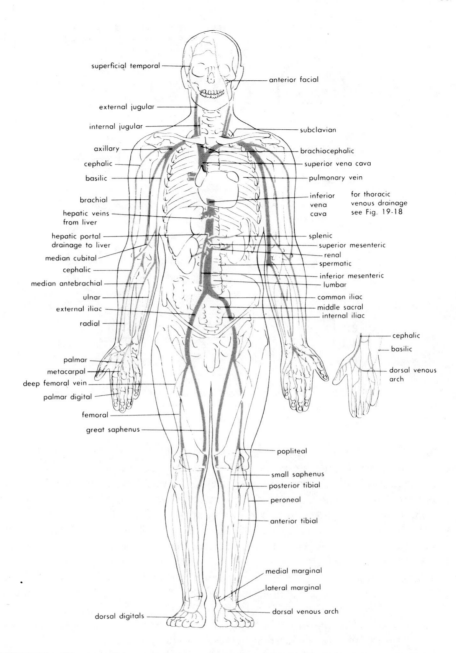

FIGURE 2. Diagram of the venous system. (From Crouch, J. E., *Functional Human Anatomy,* 3rd ed., Lea & Febiger, Philadelphia, 1978, 448. With permission.)

to the vessel size and the task of each specific segment in the arterial tree. The proportions of four of these components (leaving out the ground substance) for various sizes of arteries and veins are described in Figure 3.

The largest variation is found in the proportional amounts of collagen and elastin fibers, which are the dominant elastic materials, with smooth muscle playing the third role. It is not intended, within this text, to provide a full description of the structure and biochemistry of these components. However, to understand the different performances of various vessels it is necessary to give a short summary on the properties of these materials. The mechanical properties are to be considered later in the text.

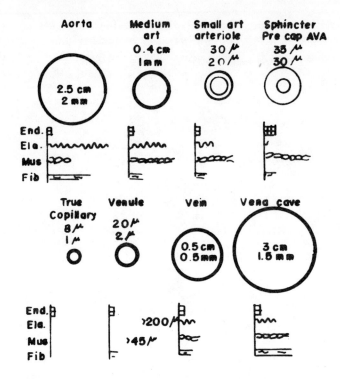

FIGURE 3.   Properties of vessel wall components in the various size of arteries and veins, and their wall to lumen diameter ratios. (From Burton, A. C., *Physiol. Rev.*, 34, 619, 1944. With permission.)

Endothelial Lining — This is the innermost layer of the vessel wall that comes in contact with the flowing blood. As such it has two major tasks. The competability to blood to prevent adhesion of various species to the vessel wall, and the selective permeability to substances such as water, electrolytes, sugars, and others that pass from the flowing blood through the vessels wall and into the tissue. It comprises of a layer of single cells, which are aligned with the direction of blood flow. From a mechanical point of view this thin layer (0.1 to 0.5 μm) has no effect on the overall elastic properties of the blood vessel.

Collagen Fibers — It is a protein substance that appears in blood vessels as strings of fibers with a serpentine shape, and a certain degree of slackness. Because of this shape they affect the mechanical properties of the blood vessels only after some stretching is achieved. The quantity of collagen in blood vessels increases with age, which is partially responsible for the increase in elastic modulus with age.

Elastin Fibers — It is also a protein substance, but very different from collagen. It has a very low resistance to stretching, but a very high expansion capability. Mechanically they behave very similar to rubber, and also their structure of long protein molecules with covalent cross-linkages resembles that of vulcanized rubber. Its higher concentration in vessels that undergo higher pulsations, points to its significance in providing the necessary circumferential strength to the blood vessels.

Smooth Muscles — Smooth muscle appears in blood vessels in two geometrical forms, longitudinal and serpentine-like shape around the vessel. The latter shape is more important as it is responsible for the vasomotor action. By contraction of this helical shape smooth muscle the tube diameter decreases (vasoconstriction). Since they are prestretched they are capable by relaxation to create a vasodilation (which increases tube cross section). The control of this kind of action is done by nerve impulses through chemical stimulation. An important function of this muscle is in the prevention of blood loss and arterial rupture in cases of local trauma. When local trauma occurs the muscle will go into spasm thus reducing the lumen diameter and thus reduce blood flow to the injured segment. The smaller cross section also helps the blood vessel to withstand the high blood pressure without rupture.

Ground Substance — Composed of nonprotein components, mainly mucopolysaccharides, that fill the spaces between the otber elements and serves as a cement agent. It also plays a major role in lubrication as well as serves as a filter and ion exchange medium. Very little is known about its mechanical properties, but it is generally assumed that they do not contribute to the overall mechanical properties of blood vessels.

The relative proportions of these substances vary with many factors, but mainly with age, see for example the section by Kirk in Abramson's book.[1]

These components are arranged in three layers. The tunica intima consists of a single layer of endothelium with a thin layer of elastin and collagen fibers. The tunica media, which forms the large part of the wall of the vessel and consists of tight helix fibers with the smooth muscle cells lying between them, and the adventitia which consists of elastin and collagen fibers that merge with the surrounding tissues. There is also a very small blood vessel, the vesa vesarum, that supplies the arterial wall.

C. Dynamic Behavior of Elastic Material

When force is applied to a material without displacing it, a relative movement of various parts of this material relative to other will occur. This relative motion is called deformation. If after the removal of the force the deformation disappears and the material regains its original shape, the material is called perfectly elastic. If after the removal of the force some deformation still remains the material is said to be plastic. The relation between the force and the deformation depends on the size of material, the magnitude of the force, and the rate with which the force is applied. To eliminate the size of the material from the calculations, there is a reference to force per unit of perpendicular area, known as stress. From this definition it is clear that stress is associated with a direction and a plane, and hence must be a tensor.

The deformation is measured relative to a determined reference situation, usually the undeformed state. However, in biological materials this undeformed, or relaxed, state is very hard to define, since all biological materials, and blood vessels in particular, are prestretched. Hence, the assumption on the exact reference situation must be defined before carrying out any measurement or analytical consideration. Unfortunately, not all the published results were done with the same reference system, and one has to be very careful in studying these results. The ratio between the deformation of a given parameter and the preload value of this parameter is called strain. Since it is a nondimensional quantity that involve stresses it is a nondimensional tensor.

If the material is perfectly elastic, and the forces are not too high, the relations between stress and strain will be linear and independent of the rate with which the force is acting. This linear relation is called Hooke's law, and the material is called Hookean solid. On the other extreme, when a force is applied to a fluid, the resulted motion of one particle relative to another will depend on the rate with which the force acts, and the viscosity of the fluid. Some material exhibits both of these properties and hence, classified as viscoelastic materials. The blood vessels are known to be of this kind, and are therefore viscoelastic. However, because of their ability to undergo large deformation they are sometimes referred to as elastomers.

Since stress and strain are tensors, and are associated with a direction, the ratio between them must also involve a specific direction. If this ratio is the same for all directions the material is said to be isotropic. If the material is isotropic and is of uniform structure it is classified as homogenous.

To define characteristic parameters, or properties, of an elastic material consider a simple case where only longitudinal stress exists. It is well known that a material stretched in one direction will undergo volume changes, and hence, size changes in the other directions. If a specimen of initial dimensions ℓ_o, a_o, b_o, are stretched to a final dimension ℓ_1, a_1, b_1, the strains can be defined by the following relations:

$$\epsilon_1 = \frac{\ell_1 - \ell_0}{\ell_0}$$

$$\epsilon_2 = \frac{a_1 - a_0}{a_0} = -\nu_2 \, \epsilon_1 \tag{1}$$

$$\epsilon_3 = \frac{b_1 - b_0}{b_0} = -\nu_3 \, \epsilon_1$$

where the ratio between the traverse and longitudinal stresses, introduced here by ν, is called the Poisson's ratio. It is obvious that in a nonisotropic material these ratios are not necessarily equal. Thus there are six independent Poisson's ratios that are characteristic of the material properties. In isotropic material all six of these parameters are equal.

If a cube of infinitesimal length is placed with the faces parallel to the coordinate axes, and an arbitrary force is applied, there will be nine stresses and nine strains components which are denoted by:

$$\epsilon_{xx}, \epsilon_{xy}, \epsilon_{xz}, \epsilon_{yx}, \epsilon_{yy}, \epsilon_{yz}, \epsilon_{zx}, \epsilon_{zy}, \epsilon_{zz}$$

$$\sigma_{xx}, \sigma_{xy}, \sigma_{xz}, \sigma_{yx}, \sigma_{yy}, \sigma_{yz}, \sigma_{zx}, \epsilon_{zy}, \epsilon_{zz}$$

Where the first subscript describing the plane and the second subscript is the direction associated with this plane, Figure 4. It can be proven that these two tensors must be symmetrical, namely:

$$\epsilon_{ij} = \epsilon_{ji} \tag{2}$$

and hence only six of the parameters are unknown.

If a tensile strain, ϵ_x, is applied to this infinitesimal cube the new dimensions of the cube can be calculated, to give:

$$x_1 = x_0 \, (1 + \epsilon_{xx})$$

$$y_1 = y_0 \, (1 - \nu_{yx} \, \epsilon_{xx}) \tag{3}$$

$$Z_1 = Z_0 \, (1 - \nu_{zx} \, \epsilon_{xx})$$

Since the cube is infinitesimal in length, and assuming small deformation, the cube can be considered orthogonal. Thus the new volume is given by:

$$\frac{\Delta V}{V_0} = \frac{V_1 - V_0}{V_0} = \epsilon_{xx} \, (1 - \nu_{yx} - \nu_{zx}) \tag{4}$$

In an isotropic material all the Poisson's ratios are the same, and Equation 4 will become:

$$\frac{\Delta V}{V_0} = \epsilon_{xx} \, (1 - 2\nu) \tag{5}$$

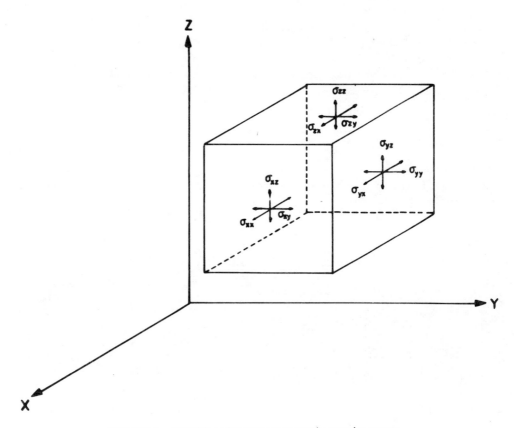

FIGURE 4.   Definition of stress components in cartesian system.

where v is Poisson's ratio for isotropic material. When the material is also incompressible, the change in volume must equal zero, and hence for such a material $v = 0.5$.

In the general case, when both stress and strain have six independent components, there can be 36 different ratios between stress and strain. However, it can be shown that 15 of them will depend on the rest. Hence, in a nonisotropic material there are 21 independent ratios, or more precisely 21 independent constants or moduli of the material. In an isotropic material they are reduced to two. To further define some of the most commonly used characteristic parameters it is useful to consider the case of isotropic material.

The ratio between longitudinal stress and the extension per unit length in this direction is defined as the Young's modulus of the material, denoted by E.

$$E = \frac{\sigma_{xx}}{\epsilon_{xx}} \tag{6}$$

The relation between the shear stress (σ_{xy}) and the angular strain ϵ_{xy} is defined as the shear modulus, G.

$$G = \frac{\sigma_{xy}}{\epsilon_{xy}} \tag{7}$$

The ratio between the average stress along the major axes and the volumetric strain is defined as the bulk modulus, K. In the case of hydrostatic pressure, the stresses in all direction and the average stress are all equal. Thus the bulk modulus can be defined as the ratio between the hydrostatic compressive force and the volumetric strain:

$$K = \frac{P}{3\frac{\Delta V}{V}} = \frac{\sigma_{xx}}{3\left(\epsilon_{xx} + \epsilon_{yy} + \epsilon_{zz}\right)} \tag{8}$$

which gives:

$$K = \frac{E}{3(1 - 2\nu)} \tag{9}$$

As was said before two parameters are sufficient, in isotropic material to describe all the characteristic parameters, as they are related to each other by the following relations:

$$E = 2(1 + \nu) \quad G = \frac{9KG}{3K + G} \tag{10}$$

$$G = \frac{E}{2(1 + \nu)} \tag{11}$$

$$K = \frac{E}{3(1 - 2\nu)} = \frac{2(1 + \nu)G}{3(1 - 2\nu)} \tag{12}$$

$$\nu = \frac{3K - 2G}{2(3K + G)} \tag{13}$$

When the material in addition to being isotropic is also incompressible we obtain:

$$\nu = 0.5; \quad E = 3G; \quad K \longrightarrow \infty \tag{14}$$

and only one parameter is sufficient to determine this material.

It is simpler in certain cases to study the dynamic behavior of an isotropic elastic material by the analogy to a combination of springs and dashpots arranged in series and in parallel. Where the spring represents pure elastic component, and the dashpot represents viscous components. The spring has a linear relation between the tension T and the strain

$$T = E \cdot \frac{\Delta \ell}{\ell} \tag{15}$$

The dashpot, is a piston moving in a fluid-filled cylinder, with fluid viscosity μ. There is a linear relation between the tension and the rate of elongation, with viscosity as the proportional coefficient:

$$T = \mu \frac{d(\Delta \ell)}{dt} \tag{16}$$

They can be arranged in series, Figure 5a which is a Maxwell body, or by a Voigt body where the arrangement is in parallel, Figure 5b.

For the series arrangement tension on both segments must be the same, and the total elongation is equal to the sum of each segmental elongation.

$$T = E \frac{\Delta \ell_1}{\ell_1} = \eta \frac{a(\Delta \ell_2)}{dt}$$

$$\Delta \ell = \Delta \ell_1 + \Delta \ell_2 \tag{17}$$

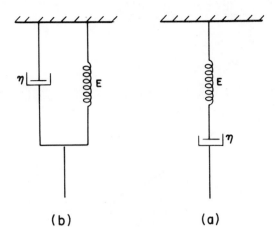

FIGURE 5. Schematic diagram of viscoelastic analog models. (a) Maxwell body; (b) Voigt body.

When a sudden elongation is applied to this system, only the spring will react by immediate stretching, giving rise to a tension equal to $E(\Delta\ell_1/\ell_1)$. After a certain period of time the dashpot will react by stretching to carry all of the springs elongation. Such a material is known as an elastic liquid, and cannot maintain a stress. The stress-time diagram of this Maxwell body is described in Figure 6.

In the parallel arrangement the conditions are reversed. The elongation is equal, and the stress is divided into the part carried by the spring and another carried by the dashpot. Because of the dashpot the system does not respond immediately, but will creep to its final value of prescribed extension. The equations are

$$T_1 = E\frac{\Delta\ell}{\ell_0}$$

$$T_2 = \mu\frac{d(\Delta\ell)}{dt} \tag{18}$$

$$T = T_1 + T_2$$

From which, the following differential equation is obtained:

$$T = E\frac{\Delta\ell}{\ell_0} + \mu\frac{d(\Delta\ell)}{dt} \tag{19}$$

and the solution, with initial condition of $\Delta\ell = 0$ is

$$\frac{\Delta\ell}{\ell_0} = \frac{T}{E}\left[1 - \exp\left(-\frac{Et}{\mu}\right)\right] \tag{20}$$

A typical response is shown in Figure 7.

Various other combinations can be considered. The most popular model for a living system is a Voigt model in series with a spring. Although, these models are very crude and not accurate, they can be found throughout the literature, mainly for their simplicity, and the easier interpretation of experimental results in creep and relaxation tests.

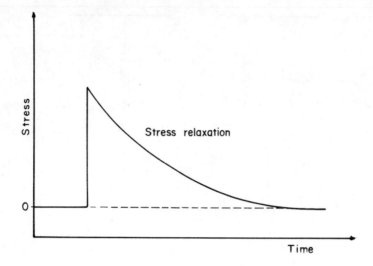

FIGURE 6.   Stress-time diagram for Maxwell body.

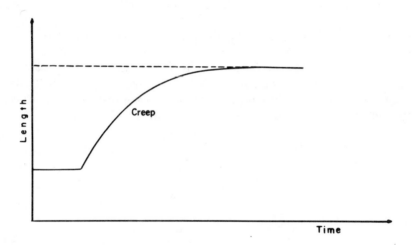

FIGURE 7.   Length-time diagram for Voigt body.

The analysis so far considered a force acting in one direction with the appropriate strains resulting from this force only. In the general case the force and, hence, stress will be in an arbitrary direction. Hence Equation 1 in the general case, will involve the effects of normal stresses in other directions:

$$\epsilon_{xx} = \frac{\sigma_{xx}}{E} - \frac{\nu\,\sigma_{yy}}{E} - \frac{\nu\,\sigma_{zz}}{E}$$

$$\epsilon_{yy} = -\frac{\nu\,\sigma_{xx}}{E} + \frac{\sigma_{yy}}{E} - \frac{\nu\,\sigma_{zz}}{E} \qquad (21)$$

$$\epsilon_{zz} = -\frac{\nu\,\sigma_{xx}}{E} - \frac{\nu\,\sigma_{yy}}{E} + \frac{\sigma_{zz}}{E}$$

The shear strains are related to the shear stresses by the shear modulus

$$\epsilon_{xy} = \frac{\sigma_{xy}}{2G}$$

$$\epsilon_{xz} = \frac{\sigma_{xz}}{2G} \tag{22}$$

$$\epsilon_{yz} = \frac{\sigma_{yz}}{2G}$$

This equation, known as the constitutive equation for isotropic solid, can be written by replacing the Young's modulus by another parameter, λ, which together with the shear modulus G are known as the Lame constants. The other moduli are related to this new parameter by the following relations:

$$\nu = \frac{\lambda}{2(\lambda + G)}$$

$$E = \frac{G(3\lambda + 2G)}{\lambda + G} \tag{23}$$

Obviously there is a requirement that $3\lambda + 2G \neq 0$. Inserting Equation 23 into Equations 21 and 22, and using summation convention, the following general equation is obtained:

$$\epsilon_{ij} = \frac{-\lambda \delta_{ij}}{2G(3\lambda + 2G)} \sigma_{nn} + \frac{1}{2G} \sigma_{ij} \tag{24}$$

where δ_{ij} is the Kronecker delta, defined by:

$$\delta_{ij} = 1 \quad \text{when } i = j \text{ and,}$$

$$\delta_{ij} = 0 \quad \text{when } i \neq j \tag{25}$$

and the summation convention which means that whenever a subscript is repeated in any of the terms, it represents summation over the range 1, 2, and 3, that stands here for x, y, and z. Thus:

$$\sigma_{nn} = \sigma_{11} + \sigma_{22} + \sigma_{33} = \sigma_{xx} + \sigma_{yy} + \sigma_{zz} \tag{26}$$

Equation 24 can be solved to give the stresses in term of the strain to yield:

$$\sigma_{ij} = 2G\epsilon_{ij} + \lambda\delta_{ij}\epsilon_{ij} \tag{27}$$

This is the general stress-strain equation for isotropic material. The strain is usually defined in terms of displacement. It can be shown to be related to displacement by the following relations:

$$\epsilon_{ij} = \frac{1}{2}\left(\frac{\partial u_i}{\partial x_j} + \frac{\partial u_j}{\partial x_i}\right) \tag{28}$$

Both stress and strain are in the general case functions of the coordinates. They must however fulfill equilibrium of forces. The forces acting on a volume element are both surface and body forces. Consider the volume element shown in Figure 6 and writing the equilibrium conditions along ox, axis, one obtains:

$$\iiint_v F_1 \, dv + \iint_s \sigma_{n_1} \, ds = 0 \tag{29}$$

where F_1 is the component of the forces in the ox, direction, σ_{n_1} are the normal stresses in the ox, direction. Writing this equation in the following form:

$$\iiint_v F_1 \, dv + \iint_s (\ell_1 \, \sigma_{11} + \ell_2 \, \sigma_{21} + \ell_3 \, \sigma_{31}) \, ds = 0 \tag{30}$$

where ℓ_1, ℓ_2, ℓ_3 are the cosine angles, enables the use of the divergence theorem to obtain the following equation:

$$\iiint_v \left[F_1 + \frac{\partial \sigma_{11}}{\partial x_1} + \frac{\partial \sigma_{21}}{\partial x_2} + \frac{\partial \sigma_{31}}{\partial x_3} \right] dv = 0 \tag{31}$$

which gives

$$F_1 + \frac{\partial \sigma_{11}}{\partial x_1} + \frac{\partial \sigma_{21}}{\partial x_2} + \frac{\partial \sigma_{31}}{\partial x_3} = 0 \tag{32}$$

The same procedure can be repeated for the other direction, to obtain the general equilibrium conditions.

$$\frac{\partial \sigma_{ij}}{\partial x_j} + F_i = 0 \tag{33}$$

In the case where the element is in motion the right hand side has to equal $\varrho \, A_1$. However, this is not appropriate to the case of cardiovascular dynamics.

The stress-strain relations, Equation 27, can be combined with the equilibrium equation, 33, to give the following equation:

$$G \, \Delta^2 \, U_i + (\lambda + G) \, \frac{\gamma \epsilon_{nn}}{\partial x_i} + F_i = 0 \tag{34}$$

These equations are known as the Navier Equations of Elasticity that are a set of differential equations whose solution will give the description of the displacement field. A use of these equations is to be discussed later in the text.

D. Mechanical Properties of the Vessel Wall Components

It is obvious from the preceding section that the analytical evaluation of vessel walls performance must consider the vessel as a composite material. This requires a description of the interaction between wall components in the process of carrying a load. However, it is well known that elastin, collagen, and smooth muscle play a role in the mechanical performance of the wall of the vessel only at certain stages of load carrying and only in specific ways. Hence, before discussing the overall properties of the vessel wall as a composite material it is necessary to consider the mechanical properties of each of the components.

The endothelial layer plays no significant role in determining the mechanical properties of the wall, since its task is to provide a smooth surface at the blood wall interface and to offer selective and controlled permeability. Hence, the mechanical properties of this monocell layer can be omitted from the discussion on overall elastic performance.

The elastin fibers are a rubbery material, and are very extensible. They are stretched 5 to 10 times more easily than rubber, Hass.[13] In stretching of up to about 60% their original length the elastin fibers follow Hooks' law. However, at extension beyond this value they will become highly nonlinear.[8] Because of this they are referred to as being a non-Hookean material. The range of Young's modulus of the elastin fibers is 3×10^6 to 6×10^6 dyn/cm², with maximum extension from 100 to 300% and with very little incremental rise in elastic moduli. The elastin fibers are the sole elastic mechanism of the arterial wall at low pressure (approximately below 60 mmHg).[15] That results in small diameter increase. At higher pressures there is a larger circumferential extension of the material of the wall and there is a recruitment of collagen that results in an increase in wall stiffness and a limit to further extension.[2,20,22] It can be concluded that elastin plays a major role in the small displacement of the arterial wall that is associated with pulsation. When this displacement gets to be large the collagen fibers will take over and dominate the performance of the wall.

Collagen is regarded as a structural component in various kinds of living tissues. Its geometry usually defines its mechanical properties. In tendons, for example, collagen is found in straight parallel bundles that result in very strong and inelastic performance; while in the heart leaflet collagen is arranged in very thin sheets that result in highly flexible properties. In the arterial wall the role of collagen is to maintain the vessel walls in steady tension, which requires a higher resistance to stretch. However, it is essential that at small displacement of the vessel wall the collagen fibers will not interfere. This is achieved by the serpentine shape of the fibers. That will permit a certain amount of radial extension and very small longitudinal extension. Although the fibers are built to withstand stretching they have a maximum extension of 50%, above this value the additional stretch can cause an irreversible damage. The behavior of collagen is non-Hookean, and exhibits some plastic deformation. The most commonly used value for its Young's modulus is 3.10^6 dyn/cm² for 100% elongation, and the average tensile strength is 1×10^8 dyn/cm². The range of values for these properties are given in Table 1.

Smooth muscles have more effect on the geometrical cross section of the arterial walls that on its mechanical properties. In the passive state they act more like a viscous fluid and less like a viscoelastic solid,[6] and thus contribute very little to the total elastic tension in the wall. However, under sympathetic stimulation they can change the vessel diameter by = (10 to 20)% in the elastic vessels,[9] and can constrict the smaller muscular vessels, even up to a total closure of the lumen.[23] Tension in the smooth muscles that causes this vasomotor action is stimulated by many mechanisms, as is shown in Table 2. For example, epinephrine is usually administered to asthma patients to decrease the size of blood vessels in the lung, so there will be more alveolar space for airflow.

The Young's modulus of smooth muscle varies from 6.10^4 dyn/cm² in the passive state to 5.10^8 dyn/cm² in the active state. In both passive and active state the maximum extension of smooth muscle is about 300%.

E. The Elastic Properties of the Arterial Wall as a Composite Material

Two different types of experiment can be employed to study the mechanical properties of blood vessel walls. The classical stress-strain test can be performed on an isolated segment of vessel wall. The results of this test depend very strongly on the

Table 1
ELASTIC PROPERTIES OF THE VESSEL WALL COMPONENTS

	Young's modulus in 100% elongation (dyn/cm²)		Tensile strength (dyn/cm²)		Maximum extension (%)	
	Range	Normal value	Range	Normal value	Range	Normal value
Collagen fibers	$1.10^9 - 3.10^9$	2.10^9	$5.10^7 - 5.10^9$	1.10^8	$5 - 50$	30
Elastin fibers	$3.10^9 - 6.10^9$	—	—	—	$100 - 200$	160
Smooth muscle	—	—	—	—	—	—
Relaxed	—	6.10^4	—	—	—	300
Contracted	$1.10^5 - 12.10^6$	1.10^6	—	—	—	300

Table 2
FACTORS THAT DETERMINE TENSION IN THE SMOOTH MUSCLE IN THE ARTERIOLES

Tension Increases with:

1. Increasing fiber length
2. Decreasing temperature (cold)
3. Increasing concentration of "vasoconstrictor" Substances such as:
   a. Epinephrine (in most vessels)
   b. Norepinephrine
   c. Angiotensin
   d. Vasopressin
   e. Vasoconstrictor drugs
4. Nervous effects

Tension Decreases with:

1. Decreasing fiber length
2. Increasing temperature (warmth)
3. Increasing concentration of "vasodilator" Substances such as:
   a. Acetylcholine $C_7H_{17}O_3N$
   b. Epinephrine (in muscle only)
   c. Metabolic (especially CO_2)
   d. Estrogens (chiefly in reproduction organs)
   e. Vasodilator drugs
4. Nervous effects

way the segment was cut. It is possible to load the segment longitudinally or radially, which will give different characteristics and will also depend on the clamping of the segment. The other type of test treats the vessel as a cylinder with variable internal pressure. The axial and tangential stresses are either measured or calculated from radial expansion measurements for various values of internal pressure. This pressure can be static or vary with time according to prescribed patterns. It is obvious that these two tests supply different kinds of information and the relation between these types of information must be obtained by a detailed analysis of the behavior of an elastic tube under distending pressure, which is the topic of the next section.

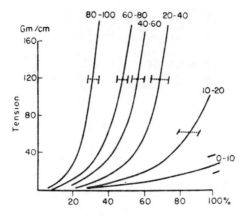

FIGURE 8. Tension in the blood vessel wall as a function of stretch, and the effect of age. (From Burton, A. C., *Physiol. Rev.*, 34, 619, 1944. With permission.)

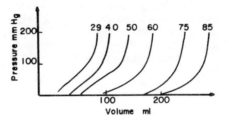

FIGURE 9. Pressure-volume diagram of human thoracic aorta. The numbers refer to age of the aortas. (From Bader, H., *Circ. Res.*, 20, 354, 1967. With permission.)

It is, however, important to summarize published results on the behavior of blood vessel wall under both types of experiments. It is expected, because the collagenous fibers are not prestretched, that the first part of the extension will be achieved with very little force. Thus for moderate stresses the overall modulus of elasticity will be very close to that of elastin fibers. It is only after a certain amount of stretching that collagen fibers play a role in the extension mechanism, and then a very sharp rise in elasticity is expected. Figure 8 shows that this is truly the case. The figure also shows that the sharp rise due to collagen interaction comes earlier with an increase in age, which corresponds to a decrease with age in the elastin/collagen ratio. The same changes with age are obtained in the second type of experiment, as was reported by Bader,[5] and shown in Figure 9. Armeniades et al.[4] showed that these changes are actually due to the elastin-collagen composition. In their results, Figure 10, they measured the stress-deformation data on a bovine aortic tissue specimen comparing the native state (A), and the cases where lipids (B), collagen (C), and elastin (D) were removed prior to performance of the tests. It also shows the different data for longitudinally and circumferentially oriented specimens. The same results were also reported by Roach and Burton,[20] Wolinsky and Glagov,[22] Goto and Kimoto,[11] and Apter,[2] as was reported in the previous section. The relations between the transverse and longitudinal strains are given by the Poisson ratio. This ratio depends on the composition of the material, and since the arterial walls are composed of 70% water the Poisson ratio has to be very close to that of water. And indeed this value is usually

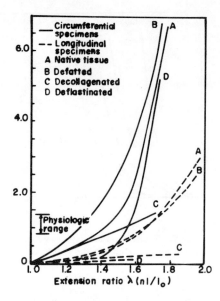

FIGURE 10. Stress-deformation data for
native, degatted, and decollagenated bovin
aortic tissue. (From Armeniades, C. O.,
Lake, L. W., Missirlis, Y. F., and Kennedy,
J. H., *Appl. Polym. Symp.*, 22, 319, 1973.
With permission.)

taken as 0.5, which corresponds to an incompressible material. This was suggested by
McDonald[16] and later confirmed by Carew, Vaishnav, and Patel[7] that showed that the
extension is truly without a change in volume.

Hartung[12] explained the second phase of stress-strain relation by using thermody-
namic principles. He used the Helmholtz free energy to show that this second phase is
caused by the "mechanical interplay of tissue elements, smooth muscle, collagen elastin, and a nonfibrous matrix, the ground substance".

The experiment carried out on arterial segments showed evidence of viscoelastic behavior. These properties are usually characterized by relaxation parameters and creep
properties. Experiments were performed to measure stress relaxation[11,17] and creep.[21]
However, the results of these experiments can be explained purly by viscoelastic properties, as there is a strong dependence on the history of strain. Thus resembling nonlinear behavior of materials with memory. It also depends heavily on the exact method
of the attachment of the stress or strain transducers. An example for this difference is
in the two reports by Patel et al.[18,19] The results of these experiments confirmed that
the shear modulus is of very little importance in distending the vascular blood vessels
and can be ignored, thus leading to an elastic symmetrical structure.

Further tests to confirm the viscoelasticity in arteries were performed by sinusoidally
applied force in both in vitro[3,14] and in vivo.[10] It can be concluded from these experiments that the more "mascular" is the blood vessel the more prominent is the viscous
effect.

Another effect which is of extreme importance but is very hard to measure is the
attachment of the various blood vessels to the surroundings. In the larger arteries this
attachment is achieved by the merging of adventitia with surrounding tissues as well
by structural complex of vessel branches. In the venous system the tissue effect is more
prominent, and because of low internal pressure the surrounding pressure might alter
significantly the transmural pressure. This might result from changes in the intrathor-

acic or intraabdominal pressure which effect total area, from intramuscular forces which effect single blood vessels or by interstitial fluid pressure in the connective tissues which effect local areas of single blood vessels.

F. The Behavior of an Elastic Tube Under a Distending Pressure

In the experiment described in the last section the response of segment of the vascular blood vessels to various forms of internal pressure were measured. To relate these measurements to characteristic parameters it is essential to obtain an analytical solution for the strains and stresses associated with either static or pulsatile internal pressure. Some of the measurements are based on the changes in speed of propagation of elastic waves, to be considered later on when the interrelation of wall displacement and flow are to be discussed. In the following analysis the flow within the vessels are ignored, and only the behavior of blood vessels under prescribed internal pressure $P_i(t)$ is being considered.

It is possible to start this discussion with the Navier's Equation 34. However, this equation already assumes isotropic material and very small deformation so that the stress-strain relations are linear. Since the geometry of the problem is well defined, and is symmetrical, it is possible to obtain the governing equations for the more general case and to subtract the solution for small deformation as a special case.

Consider a cylindrical elastic tube with inner radius R_i and outer radius of R_o. The inside of the tube is subjected to a controlled prescribed pressure $P_i(t)$, while the pressure outside of tube, P_o, is given by the surrounding pressure, which can be described by external pressure or interstitial fluid pressure in surrounding tissues. The pressure difference across the wall, $P_i - P_o$, is defined as the transmural pressure. It is assumed that the material of the wall of the vessel is incompressible and that the only displacement is in the radial direction, u_r.

When an infinitesimal segment of the vessel wall is isolated, the forces acting on this element must be in equilibrium. The net radial component associated with the radial stress is given by:

$$(\sigma_{rr} \cdot r d\theta dz)_r - (\sigma_{rr} \cdot r d\theta dz)_{r + dr} \simeq -\frac{\partial}{r} (r\sigma_{rr}) dr d\theta dz$$

The circumferential stresses have a force component along the radial direction. To obtain the value of this force it is assumed that the circumferential stress can be calculated on the bisector of the angle $d\theta$. The net result in the radial direction is

$$2 \sigma_{\theta\theta} \sin \frac{d\theta}{2} dr dz$$

which for small angles $d\theta$, can be approximated by:

$$2 \sigma_{\theta\theta} \frac{d\theta}{2} dr dz = \sigma_{\theta\theta} dr d\theta dz$$

The external force provides the acceleration associated with wall displacement, and can be obtained by Newton's second law. The element mass is given by the product of its volume given by $rdrd\theta dz$ and its density, ϱ_w, which is assumed constant. The acceleration is given by the second time derivative of the radial displacement. This results in external force given by:

$$-\rho_w r dr d\theta dz \cdot \frac{\partial^2 u_r}{\partial t^2}$$

Collecting all the terms and dividing by $drd\theta dz$, results in the following differential equation:

$$\rho_w \frac{\partial^2 u_r}{\partial t^2} = \frac{1}{r} \frac{\partial}{\partial r} (r\sigma_{rr}) - \frac{\sigma_{\theta\theta}}{r} \tag{35}$$

This equation has to be solved subject to the boundary condition of matching pressures and radial stress at the interfaces, namely:

$$\sigma_{rr} = -P_i \quad @ \quad r = R_i$$
$$\sigma_{rr} = -P_o \quad @ \quad r = R_o \tag{36}$$

A solution to this problem can be found in Love[26] (Article 100) for the isotropic case, and in Middleman[27] for the unisotropic case with zero external pressure. Consider here the case of unisotropy with given internal and external pressures. The relation between radial displacement and stresses is thus given by:

$$\sigma_{rr} = E_r \cdot \epsilon_{rr} = E_r \cdot \frac{\partial u_r}{\partial r}$$
$$\sigma_{\theta\theta} = E_\theta \cdot \epsilon_{\theta\theta} = E_\theta \cdot \frac{u_r}{r^2} \tag{37}$$

where E_r and E_θ are the radial and circumferential elastic moduli, respectively. The deviation of their ratio from the value of 1 can serve as a description of the unisotropy. Inserting Equation 37 into Equation 35, and dividing the equation by E_r gives:

$$\frac{\rho_w}{E_r} \cdot \frac{\partial^2 u_r}{\partial t^2} = \frac{1}{r} \frac{\partial}{\partial r} \left(r \frac{\partial u_r}{\partial r} \right) - \frac{E_\theta}{E_r} \cdot \frac{u_r}{r^2} \tag{38}$$

For a steady state, or for a constant internal pressure the left hand side of Equation 38 vanishes, and the partial derivative with respect to time is replaced by the regular derivative. For simplicity the ratio E_θ/E_r, the degree of unisotropy, is replaced by:

$$e^2 = E_\theta/E_r \tag{39}$$

Thus the differential equation for the radial displacement is given by:

$$\frac{1}{r} \frac{d}{dr} \left(r \frac{du_r}{dr} \right) - e^2 \frac{u_r}{r^2} = 0 \tag{40}$$

The general solution of this equation is given by:

$$u_r = C_1 r^e + C_2 r^{-e} \tag{41}$$

When subjected to the boundary condition Equation 36, the constant C_1 and C_2 are obtained:

$$C_1 = \frac{P_i R_i^{1+e} - P_o R_o^{1+e}}{E_r \cdot e (R_o^{2e} - R_i^{2e})}$$

$$C_2 = \frac{P_i R_i^{1+e} R_o^{2e} - P_o R_o^{1+e} R_i^{2e}}{E_r \cdot e (R_o^{2e} - R_i^{2e})}$$

(42)

The circumferential stress, given by Equation 37, can be calculated to give:

$$\sigma_{\theta\theta}\Big|_{r=R_o} = e \left\{ \frac{2 P_i R_o^{e-1} R_i^{1+e} - P_o (R_o^{2e} + R_i^{2e})}{R_o^{2e} - R_i^{2e}} \right\}$$

(43)

It is important to point out that even if the transmural pressure is zero, namely $P_i = P_o$, the vessel wall will still have stresses, which is in contrary to widely spread consent among physiologist that the vessel is unstressed when the transmural pressure is zero.

This stress can be measured experimentally. However, this stress and pressure are not sufficient to determine both elastic modulus. In all the experiments described in the previous section, this equation was used to calculate the apparent elastic modulus assuming the material is isotropic. The attachment of the strain gauge requires exposure of the outer surface of the vessel wall, thus eliminating the outer pressure P_o. For such a case the circumferential stress can be calculated from Equation 43 by assuming zero external pressure, leading to the following result:

$$\sigma_{\theta\theta}\Big|_{r=R_o} = \frac{2 P_i e \left(\dfrac{R_o}{R_i}\right)^{e-1}}{\left(\dfrac{R_o}{R_i}\right)^{2e} - 1}$$

(44)

By assuming $e = 1$, the circumferential stress, can be obtained:

$$\sigma_{\theta\theta}\Big|_{r=R_o} = \frac{2 P_i}{\left(\dfrac{R_o}{R_i}\right)^2 - 1}$$

(45)

The result of Equation 45 is used to calculate the apparent elastic modulus.

$$E_{app} = \frac{2 P_i}{\left(\dfrac{\Delta R}{R_o}\right)\left[\dfrac{R_o^2}{R_i^2} - 1\right]}$$

(46)

However, if there is a certain unisotropy there will be an error, ϕ, which is given by the ratio of Equations 46 and 44:

$$\phi = e \left(\frac{R_e}{R_i}\right)^{e-1} \frac{\left(\dfrac{R_o}{R_i}\right)^2 - 1}{\left(\dfrac{R_o}{R_i}\right)^{2e} - 1}$$

(47)

It is clear that there are two sources for error in the measurement of elastic modulus. One depends on the type of vascular segment used in the experiment, which will define the ratio of outer to inner radii, and the other is the degree of unisotropy. The degree of unisotropy depends on range of pressures used in the experiment. For high pressures the collagen becomes the dominated factor in the radial displacement determination, and the level of unisotropy might be very high, with e^2 reaching values as high as 100, Middleman.[27] At low pressure the dominate response is that of elastin, for which the value of e^2 is very close to 1. It should be noted that this is not the total error, since there is always the contributions of external pressure, which are very complex and cannot be introduced easily into the calculation of errors. The case corresponding to a thin wall, approach that of a membrane, for which the results approach those given by Laplace's law, described in Chapter 2.

Some experiments were carried out under conditions of pulsatile pressure. For this case some additional parameters must be considered: the frequency of pulsation and the viscoelastic parameters of the vessel wall. The viscoelastic properties, which are not visible in steady state situations, are highly important in the pulsatile case. This will not only change the amplitude of radial displacement, but will also cause a phase lag between the internal pressure and the radial displacement.

The internal pressure is assumed to be sinusoidal, given by:

$$P_i(t) = P_{io} + P_i \sin \omega t = P_{io} + R_e \left\{ \bar{P}_i e^{i\omega t} \right\} \qquad (48)$$

Since there is an assumed linearity the solution for the static pressure component can be obtained separately, as was done previously, and the pulsatile component added to this solution by superposition. Thus the pressure can be assumed to be:

$$P_i(t) = R_e \left\{ \bar{P}_i \cdot e^{i\omega t} \right\} \qquad (49)$$

The governing differential equation is given by Equation 35. It is possible, because of linearity, to assume that stresses, strains and displacement must also be of the form:

$$u_r(r,t) = R_e \left(U(r) \cdot e^{i\omega t} \right)$$

$$\sigma_{ij}(r,t) = R_e \left(\sigma_{ij}^{\star}(r) \cdot e^{i\omega t} \right) \qquad (50)$$

$$\epsilon_{ij}(r,t) = R_e \left(\epsilon_{ij}^{\star}(r) \cdot e^{i\omega t} \right)$$

Where U, $\bar{P}_i$, σ^*_{ij} and ε^*_{ij} can be complex functions. Inserting this relation into Equation 37 requires having a complex elastic moduli. The complex elastic modulus describes both solid and viscous components of the vessel wall. This is actually equivalent to assuming a first order differential equation for the stress strain relation, like:

$$\sigma_{ij} + \alpha \frac{\partial \sigma_{ij}}{\partial t} = E \left(\epsilon_{ij} + \beta \frac{\epsilon_{ij}}{\partial t} \right) \qquad (51)$$

or assuming a combination of springs and dashpots in parallel. Insertion of Equations 49 and 50 into Equation 35 results in the following equation:

$$-\frac{\rho_w}{E_r^\star} + \frac{1}{r}\frac{dU}{dr} - \frac{E_\theta^\star}{E_r^\star}\left(1 - \frac{\rho_w \cdot \omega^2}{E_\theta^\star}r^2\right)\frac{U}{r^2} = 0 \tag{52}$$

Where $E_r^\star$ and $E_\theta^\star$ are the complex elastic moduli.

The second term in parenthesis is very small, for vascular vessels, and can be either ignored, or replaced by its possible maximum value:

$$\frac{\rho_w \cdot \omega^2}{E_\theta^\star} R^2$$

This will result in a simple equation, although it is also possible to obtain a closed solution for Equation 52. Hence by defining:

$$s^2 = \left(1 - \frac{\rho_w \cdot \omega^2}{E_\theta^\star} \cdot R^2\right)\frac{E_\theta^\star}{E_r^\star} \tag{53}$$

Equation 52 becomes:

$$\frac{d^2 U}{dr^2} + \frac{1}{r}\frac{dU}{dr} - S^2 \frac{U}{r^2} = 0 \tag{54}$$

which, with S replacing e, is identical to Equation 40. Thus the previous solution can be used. It is, however, simpler to assume *a priori* that there is no external pressure, which will give the following solution:

$$u_r(r,t) = R_e\left\{\left[\frac{P\, r_i^{1+s}\cdot r^s}{E_r^\star s\,(R_o^{2s} - R_i^{2s})} + \frac{P\, R_i^{1+s}\, R_o^{2s}\, r^{-s}}{E_r^\star s\,(R_o^{2s} - R_i^{2s})}\right] e^{i\omega t}\right\} \tag{55}$$

and the circumferential stress at the outer surface is given by:

$$R_e\left\{\frac{\Delta R}{R_o} e^{i\omega t}\right\} = R_e\left\{\frac{2P}{E_r^\star s}\frac{R_o^{s-1}\cdot R_i^{s+1}}{[R_o^{2s} - R_i^{2s}]} e^{i\omega t}\right\} \tag{56}$$

Since S is a complex function, the solution cannot be obtained in a closed form. However, it is clear from these equations that there will be a time lag between radial displacement and circumferential stress, and between these two and internal pressure.

In the limit, where the second term is parenthesis in Equation 52 is neglected, and when isotropy is assumed, namely $E_\theta^* = E_r^*$, Equation 56 can be reduced to a simple form:

$$R_e\left\{\frac{\Delta R}{R_o} e^{i\omega t}\right\} = R_e\left\{\frac{2P}{E_r^\star}\frac{R_i^2}{R_o^2 - R_i^2} e^{i\omega t}\right\} \tag{57}$$

from Equation 48 one can obtain that $\overline{P}_i = iP_1$. If E_r^* can be written as a complex number Equation 57 can be used to obtain the phase difference between pressure and displacement. It can be shown by the use of Equation 51 that this complex number must be a function of frequency (because of time derivatives). Equations 50 and 51, can be used to show that stress-strain relations must be of the form:

$$(1 + \lambda_1\ i\omega)\ \sigma_{ij} = E\ (1 + \lambda_2 i\omega)\ \epsilon_{ij} \tag{58}$$

where λ_1 and λ_2 are defined as relaxation constants. Thus giving:

$$E_r^{\star} = E_\theta^{\star} = E\ \frac{1 + \lambda_2 i\omega}{1 + \lambda_1 i\omega} \tag{59}$$

which after insertion into Equation 57 gives

$$\frac{\Delta R}{R_0} = \frac{2\ P_i}{E\left[\left(\frac{R_0}{R_i}\right)^2 - 1\right]\left(1 + \omega^2\lambda_2^2\right)}\left\{\left(1 + \omega^2\lambda_1\lambda_2\right)\sin\omega t + \omega\left(\lambda_1 - \lambda_2\right)\cos\omega t\right\} \tag{60}$$

which results in a phase difference given by:

$$\psi = \tan^{-1}\frac{\omega\left(\lambda_1 - \lambda_2\right)}{1 + \omega^2\lambda_1\lambda_2} \tag{61}$$

This phase difference depends on the frequency. The phase difference, through a series of phase measurements, can give the values of these two relaxation constants.

It is also possible to incorporate nonlinear viscoelasticity into the solution. This nonlinearity is usually associated with history depended deformation, referred to as memory. This can be used to further analyze the properties of the material, but is too complex to be included in actual flow condition, and therefore is not discussed further here. Young, Vaishnav, and Patel,[29] presented theoretical analysis for the nonlinear viscoelasticity of canine aortas by assuming thick walled elastic segment which are considered incompressible and orthotropic. The stress strain relations are assumed to be described by the idea of functional, introduced by Green and Rivlin,[25] which involve four or ten relaxation functions and histories of circumferential and longitudinal strains.

REFERENCES

1. Abramson, D. I., Ed., *Blood Vessels and Lymphatics,* Academic Press, New York, 1962.
2. Apter, J. T., Correlation of visco-elastic properties with microscopic structure of large arteries. IV. Thermal responses of collagen, elastin smooth muscle and intact arteries, *Circ. Res.,* 21, 901, 1967.
3. Apter, J. T. and Marquez, E., Correlation of visco-elastic properties of large arteries with microscopic structure, *Circ. Res.,* 22, 393, 1968.
4. Armeniades, C. D., Lake, L. W., Misorilis, Y. F., and Kennedy, J. H., Histologic origin of aortic tissue mechanics: the role of collageneous and elastic structures, *Appl. Polym. Symp.,* 22, 319, 1973.
5. Bader, H., Dependence of wall stress in the human thoracic aorta on age and pressure, *Circ. Res.,* 20, 354, 1967.
6. Bergel, D. H., Arterial viscoelasticity, in *Pulsatile Blood Flow,* Attinger, E. O., Ed., McGraw-Hill, New York, 1964, 275.
7. Carew, T. E., Vaishnav, R. N., and Patel, D. J., Compressibility of the arterial wall, *Circ. Res.,* 23, 61, 1968.
8. Carton, R. W., Dainauskas, J., and Clarke, J. W., Elastic properties of single elastic fibers, *J. Appl. Physiol.,* 17, 547, 1962.
9. Gerova, M. and Gero, J., Range of the sympathetic control of the dogs femoral artery, *Circ. Res.,* 24, 349, 1969.

10. **Gow, B. S. and Taylor, M. G.,** Measurement of visco-elastic properties of arteries in the living dog, *Circ. Res.,* 23, 111, 1968.
11. **Goto, M. and Kimoto, Y.,** Hysterisis and stress relaxation of the blood vessels studied by universal tensile testing instrument, *Jpn. J. Physiol.,* 15, 169, 1966.
12. **Hartung, C.,** Vascular tissues — a two-phase material, in *Biopolymere and Biomechanik von Binde-gewbssystemen,* Hartman, F., Ed., Springer-Verlag, Basel, 1974, 211.
13. **Hass, G. M.,** Elastic Tissue. III. Relations between the structure of the aging aorta and the properties of the isolated aortic elastic tissue, *Arch. Pathol.,* 35, 29, 1943.
14. **Learoyd, B. M. and Taylor, M. G.,** Alterations with age in the visco-elastic properties of human aortic walls, *Circ. Res.,* 18, 278, 1966.
15. **Ling, S. C. and Atabek, H. B.,** A nonlinear analysis of pulsatile flow in arteries, *J. Fluid Mech.,* 55, 493, 1972.
16. **McDonald, D. A.,** Blood flow in arteries, *Monogr. Physiol. Soc. London,* Edward Arnold, London, 1960.
17. **Mikami, T. and Attinger, E. O.,** Stress relaxation of blood vessel walls, *Angiologica,* 5, 281, 1968.
18. **Patel, D. J., Greenfield, J. C., and Fry, D. L.,** In vivo pressure-length-radius relationship of certain vessels in man and dog, in *Pulsatile Blood Flow,* Attinger, E. O., Ed., McGraw–Hill, New York, 1964, 293.
19. **Patel, D. J., Janicki, J. S., and Carew, T. E.,** Static anisotropic elastic properties of the aorta in living dogs, *Circ. Res.,* 25, 765, 1969.
20. **Roach, M. R. and Burton, A. C.,** Effect of age on the elasticity of human iliac arteries, *Can. J. Biochem. Physiol.,* 37, 577, 1959.
21. **Wiederhielm, C. A.,** Distensibility characteristics of small blood vessels, *Fed. Proc.,* 24, 1075, 1965.
22. **Wolinsky, H. and Giagor, S.,** Structural basis for the static mechanical properties of the aortic media, *Circ. Res.,* 14, 400, 1964.
23. **Van Citters, R. L.,** Occlusion of lumina in small arterioles during vasconstriction, *Circ. Res.,* 18, 199, 1966.
24. **Burton, A. C.,** Relation of structure to function of the tissues of the wall of blood vessels, *Physiol. Rev.,* 34, 619, 1944.
25. **Green, A. E. and Rivlin, R. S.,** The mechanics of non-linear materials with memory. I, *Arch. Ration. Mech. Anal.,* 1, 1, 1957.
26. **Love, A. E. H.,** *A Treatise on the Mathematical Theory of Elasticity,* Dover, New York, 1927.
27. **Middleman, S.,** *Transport Phenomena in the Cardiovascular System,* Wiley-Interscience, New York, 1972.
28. **Millard, N. D. and King, B. G.,** *Human Anatomy and Physiology,* 3rd ed., W. B. Saunders, Philadelphia, 1951.
29. **Young, J. T., Vaishav, R. N., and Patel, D. J.,** Nonlinear anisotropic viscoelastic properties of canine arterial systems, *J. Biomech.,* 10, 549, 1977.

Chapter 5

PROPAGATION OF WAVES IN ARTERIES

A. Pressure Wave Profiles in the Circulatory System

Blood is ejected from the left ventricle into the circulatory system by a periodic action of the heart. This added blood creates a change in pressure and results in flow of blood along the aorta and throughout the circulatory system. At any given point the pressure and velocity will change periodically, and hence, the flow is pulsatile associated with a propagation of pressure wave. The volume ejected from the left ventricle is not constant, and might vary from one beat to another. This, together with the fact that the aortic valve does not close by a pressure difference mechanism, does not permit a clear decision on whether the heart is a "constant volume" or "constant pressure" pump, and is actually a nonuniform and nonlinear combination of both. Historically the reference was always made to blood pressure, because of the development of clinical measurement procedures. In reality, the volumetric flow rates are more important, but also harder to measure. It is mainly due to this reason: that empirical relation between blood pressure parameters and pathological conditions were developed to become one of the most useful diagnostic tools. This was developed mainly for the aorta, brachial arteries, and other large arteries in the human body. Throughout the arterial system the pressure rises to a peak value, defined as systolic pressure. In the aorta the normal value for the systolic pressure is 120 mmHg. The minimum value of the pressure pulse is defined as the diastolic pressure, and the normal value at the brachial artery is about 70 to 80 mmHg. The difference between these two extremes is defined as the pulse pressure, as this is the rise in pressure the left ventricle has to initiate. Two values are used for the average or mean pressure in the arterial system, the simple mathematical average and the mean pressure with respect to time, which require integration of the pressure curve. It can however be calculated fairly accurately by:

$$(\text{systolic} + 2\,\text{diastolic})/3 = \text{diastolic} + \frac{\text{pulse}}{3}$$

The pressure wave changes both its shape and peak value as it travels down the arterial system. The reasons for this change are many, and should be considered separately although the effects they have on the pressure wave are related to eachother and cannot be defined separately. There are two types of tapering that describe the arterial system: the geometrical tapering which is a decrease in cross-sectional area and the elastic tapering which is an increase in wall stiffness. In the medium-sized arteries the elastic tapering is very small and the pressure falls only slightly. However, in the smaller vessels both types of tapering are highly significant, and the pressure falls rapidly, reaching a mean value of 30 to 38 mmHg in the arterioles, and pulse pressure of only 5 mmHg. These values are true for regular conditions and might change drastically when the arterioles are either constricted or dilated. By the time the pressure wave reaches the capillaries, the pulsations are almost completely damped out, except in cases of marked vasodilatation. This damping is due to the viscosity of the blood and the viscous component of the viscoelastic arterial wall. In addition to the effect of increasing elastic stiffness of the arteries and the tapering there is a major additional effect associated with the branching of the arterial tree and discontinuities of elastic properties. Whenever a pressure wave reaches a branch or discontinuity part of the wave is transmitted and part of the wave is reflected. This reflection of positive pressure wave is added to original wave, and a higher amplitude might be reached at a downstream point. This increase in pressure amplitude away from the heart, called "peaking" of the pulse, depends on the amount of constriction in the arterioles, and the activity of the precapillary resistance barrier — the precapillary sphincter,[11] which might act as a closed end to the pressure wave. The reflected wave is "re-reflected" to some extent, till it damps out. The superposition of propagated and reflected pressure waves that creates the peaking of the wave also causes dispersion of the wave. The aortic pressure wave, which is triangular-shaped, becomes rounded and spread out when reaching the arterioles. The slight increase in pressure following the incisura, Figure 1, which is due to wave reflection becomes rounded and gradually replaced by slow but marked dip.[8] The mechanism of annihilation or amplification of the pressure wave is different for different components of the pulse, as the various components of the pressure wave might travel at different speeds. This velocity which can be different for the various components requires a separate discussion for each component. However, it is convenient to discuss group velocity. In most published work the treatment of the speed of propagation of the pressure wave is usually referred to this group velocity. The speed of transmission of the pulse is about 3 m/sec in the thoracic aorta and 5 or more m/sec in the smaller blood vessels where collagen predominates. Structural changes in the arterial wall greatly influence the speed of propagation. Pathological changes such as wall sclerosis or hypertension as well as muscle contraction in the arterial wall, that result in decreased distensibility of the walls, results in an increase in speed of propagation, which is closer to a rigid tube.

Additional changes in the pressure profile can happen due to centrifugal pressure gradient that occurs in flow in bend tubes, or due to occurrence of natural vibrations in various parts of the arterial tree, mainly in segments with a certain degree of stenosis. There is also an external effect of secondary pulsation due to respiration and changes in the intrathoracic pressure, and external pressure that results in changes in interstitial tissue pressure. All of these phenomena will be discussed analytically in the following chapter.

B. Pressure Flow Relation in the Circulatory System

The measurement of velocity profile in arteries and vein was not possible until the last decade without the distortion of the natural profile by introduction of instruments into the stream. Only in the last decade with the development of pulsed doppler flowmeters, is it possible to obtain velocity distribution across the blood vessels. Other techniques like tracer or electromagnetic flowmeter yield information on the average properties of flow. It is for this reason that the clinical "data bank" that was collected during the years relate the different pathological situation to deviation of pressure parameters, like systolic and diastolic blood pressure. This can explain why early analytical calculation of pressure-flow relation in the arterial system,[12] was considered a theoretical exercise and ignored for half a century. With the new measurement techniques it was realized that flow distribution and flow rates contain more clinical information, and can serve as a better diagnostic tool for the source of pathological changes, than the blood pressure.

It was only in late 1950s that researchers realized that it is the pressure gradient along the blood vessel which determines the flow conditions, especially in pulsatile flow. This pressure gradient oscillates about a mean value, but will change when traveling down the arterial tree due to the different geometry and different elastic parameter, which determine its speed of propagation. The existence of reflection sites further complicates the situation, since the positive reflected pressure wave can be associated with a negative velocity. This may explain why vasomotor activity, either vasoconstriction or vasodilation, might change the flow by an order of magnitude, while changes in blood pressure do not exceed 15 to 20%.

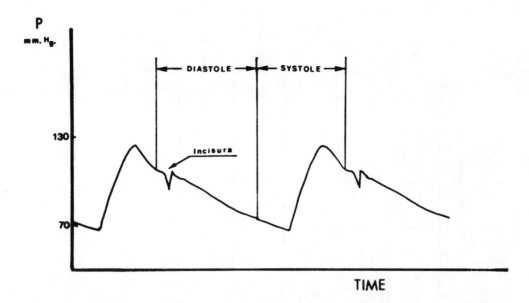

FIGURE 1.   The shape of the arterial pressure wave.

The velocity at the most part of the arterial tree is phasic. In the aorta the peak of the velocity might reach values of 100 to 150 cm/sec, under normal conditions; yet the reference is usually made to the average velocity, which in the aorta is about 40 cm/sec. The average velocity in the various part of the arterial tree can be calculated very easily by the use of continuity, as the number of vessels and typical cross section is known. Figure 2 describes the changes in average velocity as the blood flow down the systemic circulation. Although the velocity is less pulsatile in the capillaries, there is still pressure and velocity fluctuations in the venous system. This is caused mainly by the pumping action of the right atrium of the heart.

Analytical considerations of the pressure-velocity relations are very complex. In the following sections when these relations are discussed, various assumptions on the nature of either flow or pressure gradient will be used to explain various components. At the beginning, blood will be considered as a nonviscous fluid, flowing under steady state conditions without reflection and initial entry length. These assumptions will be gradually relaxed in subsequent sections.

C. Nonpulsatile Flow Equations

To start the discussion it is necessary to derive the basic relations that relate flow and fluid parameters. The first such relation is the conservation of mass. Consider an infinitesimal volume within the fluid. For simplicity this volume will be considered with sides parallel to the Cartesian coordinates, Figure 3. The accumulation of mass within this infinitesimal volume element must equal the difference between the gain and loss in mass. The velocity of the fluid can be written in Cartesian coordinates as the sum of three components, namely, the velocity vector is given by:

$$\vec{v} = v_x\hat{i} + v_y\hat{j} + v_z\hat{k} \qquad (1)$$

The accumulation of mass, in a small interval of time Δt, is given by $\Delta(\varrho\Delta x\Delta y\Delta z) = \Delta x\Delta y\Delta z\Delta\varrho$ where ϱ is the density of the fluid.

The gain in mass is due to fluid entering the volume element, while the loss in mass results from fluid leaving the element.

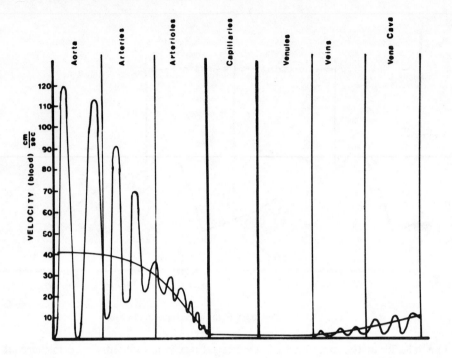

FIGURE 2. Distribution of the mean velocity of blood flow and velocity fluctuations in the various arteries and veins.

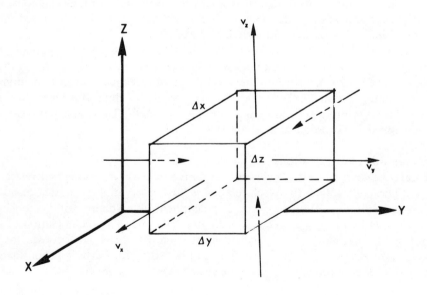

FIGURE 3. Definition of velocities in Cartesian coordinates.

	x - direction	y - direction	z - direction
Mass gain	$\varrho v_x|x \Delta y \Delta z \Delta t$	$\varrho v_y|_y \Delta x \Delta z \Delta t$	$\varrho v_z|_z \Delta x \Delta y \Delta t$
Mass loss	$\varrho v_x|_{x+\Delta x} \Delta y \Delta z \Delta t$	$\varrho v_y|_{y+\Delta y} \Delta x \Delta z \Delta t$	$\varrho_z|_{z+\Delta z} \Delta x \Delta y \Delta t$

Summing all of these changes in mass results in the following equation:

$$\Delta x \Delta y \Delta z \Delta \rho = \left(\rho v_x|_x - \rho v_x|_{x+\Delta x}\right) \Delta y \Delta z \Delta t +$$
$$\left(\rho v_y|_y - \rho v_y|_{y+\Delta y}\right) \Delta x \Delta z \Delta t +$$
$$\left(\rho v_z|_z - \rho v_z|_{z+\Delta z}\right) \Delta x \Delta y \Delta t$$

Dividing this relation by $\Delta x \Delta y \Delta z \Delta t$, and taking the limit when all of these infinitesimal value approach zero, the following relation is obtained:

$$\frac{\partial \rho}{\partial t} + \frac{\partial}{\partial x}\left(\rho v_x\right) + \frac{\partial}{\partial y}\left(\rho v_y\right) + \frac{\partial}{\partial z}\left(\rho v_z\right) = 0 \qquad (2)$$

This equation, known as the equation of continuity, can be written in the following way by using the definition of divergence:

$$\frac{\partial \rho}{\partial t} + \left(\nabla \cdot \rho \vec{v}\right) = 0 \qquad (3)$$

The second term can be expanded by:

$$\nabla \cdot \rho v = \rho\left(\nabla \cdot \vec{v}\right) + \left(\vec{v} \cdot \nabla \rho\right)$$

resulting in the following relation:

$$\frac{\partial \rho}{\partial t} + \left(\vec{v} \cdot \nabla \rho\right) + \rho\left(\nabla \cdot \vec{v}\right) = 0$$

The first two terms are usually combined into one by using the definition suggested by Euler in 1755:

$$\frac{D\rho}{Dt} = \frac{\partial \rho}{\partial t} + \left(\vec{v} \cdot \nabla \rho\right) = \frac{\partial \rho}{\partial t} + v_x \frac{\partial \rho}{\partial x} + v_y \frac{\partial \rho}{\partial y} + v_z \frac{\partial \rho}{\partial z} \qquad (4)$$

The derivative D/Dt is known as the "follow the motion" derivative, or simply the following time derivative. This equation implies that the coordinate system is moving with the material at the same velocity. The most common name for this derivative is the Lagrangian derivative, after the French mathematician that used it for this description. With this definition the equation of continuity is given by:

$$\frac{D\rho}{Dt} + \rho\left(\nabla \cdot v\right) = 0 \qquad (5)$$

When the fluid is incompressible, namely the density ϱ is constant throughout the flow field at all times this equation is reduced to:

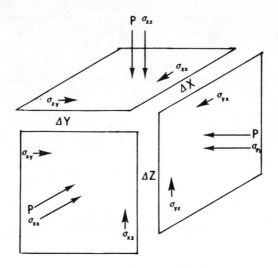

FIGURE 4.   Description of shear and normal stresses.

$$\nabla \cdot \vec{v} = \frac{\partial v_x}{\partial x} + \frac{\partial v_y}{\partial y} + \frac{\partial v_z}{\partial z} = 0 \qquad\qquad (6)$$

The assumption made in reaching this equation was that the fluid is homogeneous. This assumption will have to be changed when the various blood cells are to be considered, especially in cases of particles deposition on the vessel walls.

The other principle that must be satisfied is Newton's second law, that sum of all forces in a certain direction must equal the mass time acceleration in the same direction. This condition must be true in all three major directions; hence, the equation derived for one direction can be repeated for the other two. Consider forces and acceleration in the direction of the x-axis, for the volume element shown in Figure 4. The acceleration is given by the Lagrangian derivative of velocity component in the x direction. Hence,

$$(\rho \Delta x \Delta y \Delta z) \cdot \frac{Dv_x}{Dt} = \Sigma \,(\text{forces in x-direction})$$

The forces acting in this element are composed of pressure forces, shear forces given by shear stress times the appropriate area, normal forces and body forces. A description of the shear and normal stresses is given in Figure 4. Denote by (+) the forces acting in the positive x direction and by (−) the forces acting in the negative direction.

	(+)	(−)
Pressure forces	$(P)_x \Delta y \Delta z$	$(P)_{x+\Delta x} \Delta y \Delta z$
Shear forces	$(\sigma_{yx})_y \Delta x \Delta z$	$(\sigma_{yx})_{y+\Delta y} \Delta x \Delta z$
	$(\sigma_{zx})_z \Delta \Delta y$	$(\sigma_{zx})_{z+\Delta z} \Delta x \Delta y$
Normal forces	$(\sigma_{xx})_x \Delta y \Delta z$	$(\sigma_{xx})_{z+\Delta z} \Delta y \Delta z$
Body forces	$(\varrho \Delta x \Delta y \Delta z) g_x$	

where g_x is the component of gravity in the positive x direction. Summing up all of these terms, dividing throughout by $\Delta x \Delta y \Delta z$, and taking the limit when all of this infinitesimal length approach zero results in the following equation:

$$\rho \frac{Dv_x}{Dt} = -\frac{\partial p}{\partial x} - \left(\frac{\partial \sigma_{xx}}{\partial x} + \frac{\partial \sigma_{yx}}{\partial y} + \frac{\partial \sigma_{zx}}{\partial z}\right) + \rho g_x \qquad (7)$$

The same type of equation can be derived for the other two velocity components. These equations are known as the equations of motion.

For the case of Newtonian fluid with constant properties, the stress-strain relation, given by Equations 27 and 28 in Chapter 4 can be used to give:

$$\sigma_{xx} = -2\mu \frac{\partial v_x}{\partial x} \; ; \; \sigma_{yy} = -2\mu \frac{\partial v_y}{\partial y} \; ; \; \sigma_{zz} = -2\mu \frac{\partial v_z}{\partial z}$$

$$\sigma_{xy} = -\mu \left(\frac{\partial v_x}{\partial y} + \frac{\partial v_y}{\partial x}\right) \; ; \; \sigma_{xz} = -\mu \left(\frac{\partial v_z}{\partial x} + \frac{\partial v_x}{\partial z}\right) \qquad (8)$$

$$\sigma_{yz} = -\mu \left(\frac{\partial v_y}{\partial z} + \frac{\partial v_z}{\partial y}\right)$$

Inserting these relations into Equation 7 results in:

$$\rho \frac{Dv_x}{Dt} = -\frac{\partial p}{\partial x} + \mu \left(\frac{\partial^2 v_x}{\partial x^2} + \frac{\partial^2 v_y}{\partial y^2} + \frac{\partial^2 v_z}{\partial z^2}\right) + \rho g_x \qquad (9)$$

Equation 9 is the equation of motion for a Newtonian fluid is known as the Navier-Stokes equation. This equation, together with the equation of continuity, describe completely the flow of incompressible Newtonian fluid with constant viscosity. The left hand side of this equation, the Lagrangian derivative, contain products of the velocity component and their derivatives and therefore introduces nonlinearity. Because of this nonlinearity it is impossible to use the superposition principle, and each situation must be solved by assuming these two equations.

As most of the solutions to these equations to be presented later involve flow in cylindrical tubes, it is appropriate to use Equations 6 and 9 in cylindrical orthogonal coordinates (x, r, θ):

Equation of continuity:

$$\nabla \cdot \vec{v} = \frac{\partial u}{\partial x} + \frac{1}{r} \frac{\partial}{\partial r} (vr) + \frac{1}{r} \frac{\partial w}{\partial \theta} = 0 \qquad (10)$$

where u is the longitudinal component of the velocity, v is the radial component, and w is the circumferential component. The equations of motion, the Navier-Stokes equations, are given as:

$$\frac{\partial v}{\partial t} + v\frac{\partial v}{\partial r} + \frac{w}{r}\frac{\partial v}{\partial \theta} - \frac{v^2}{r} + u\frac{\partial v}{\partial x} = g_r - \frac{1}{\rho}\frac{\partial p}{\partial r} + \nu\left(\frac{\partial^2 v}{\partial r^2} + \frac{1}{r}\frac{\partial v}{\partial r} - \frac{v}{r^2} + \frac{1}{r^2}\frac{\partial^2 v}{\partial \theta^2}\right.$$
$$\left. - \frac{2}{r^2}\frac{\partial w}{\partial \theta} + \frac{\partial^2 v}{\partial x^2}\right)$$

$$\frac{\partial w}{\partial t} + v\frac{\partial w}{\partial r} + \frac{w}{r}\frac{\partial w}{\partial \theta} + \frac{wv}{r} + u\frac{\partial w}{\partial x} = g_\theta - \frac{1}{\rho r}\frac{\partial p}{\partial \theta} + \nu\left(\frac{\partial^2 w}{\partial r^2} + \frac{1}{r}\frac{\partial w}{\partial r} - \frac{w}{r^2} + \frac{1}{r^2}\frac{\partial^2 w}{\partial \theta^2}\right. \qquad (11)$$
$$\left. + \frac{2}{r^2}\frac{\partial v}{\partial \theta} + \frac{\partial^2 w}{\partial x^2}\right)$$

$$\frac{\partial u}{\partial t} + v\frac{\partial u}{\partial r} + \frac{w}{r}\frac{\partial u}{\partial \theta} + u\frac{\partial u}{\partial x} = g_x - \frac{1}{\rho}\frac{\partial p}{\partial x} + \nu\left(\frac{\partial^2 u}{\partial r^2} + \frac{1}{r}\frac{\partial u}{\partial r} + \frac{1}{r^2}\frac{\partial^2 u}{\partial \theta^2} + \frac{\partial^2 u}{\partial x^2}\right)$$

where ν is the kinematic viscosity.

Most of the discussion on blood flow will assume the existence of axisymmetric flow, which is characterized by w = O and $(\partial/\partial\theta)$ = O. This results in the following equations:

Continuity:

$$\frac{\partial u}{\partial x} + \frac{1}{r}\frac{\partial}{\partial r}(rv) = 0 \tag{12}$$

Navier-Stokes:

$$\frac{\partial u}{\partial t} + v\frac{\partial u}{\partial r} + u\frac{\partial u}{\partial x} = g_x - \frac{1}{\rho}\frac{\partial p}{\partial x} + \nu\left(\frac{\partial^2 u}{\partial r^2} + \frac{1}{r}\frac{\partial u}{\partial r} + \frac{\partial^2 u}{\partial x^2}\right)$$
$$\frac{\partial v}{\partial t} + v\frac{\partial v}{\partial r} + w\frac{\partial v}{\partial x} = -\frac{1}{\rho}\frac{\partial p}{\partial r} + \nu\left(\frac{\partial^2 v}{\partial r^2} + \frac{1}{r}\frac{\partial v}{\partial r} - \frac{v}{r^2} + \frac{\partial^2 v}{\partial x^2}\right) \tag{13}$$

D. Mones-Korteweg Wave Speed in Flexible Tube

Consider a segment of the artery in which blood flows, taken as an incompressible nonviscous fluid. The segment can be represented by an elastic tube of radius "a" which undergoes vibrations only in the transverse direction. The instantaneous radius of tube is described by a + η (x,t), where is assumed that the vibration are very small relative to the initial radius, namely $\eta \ll$ a. The fluid flowing in the tube is incompressible, hence the equation of continuity is given by Equation 12, where axial symmetry had been considered. Both axial and radial velocities are functions of time, in addition to being functions of the longitudinal and radial coordinates.

The average axial velocity, $\bar{u}(x,t)$, can be calculated by integration of the velocity across the tube cross section. As the assumption of small vibration was already met, this average velocity is defined by:

$$\bar{u}(x,t) = \frac{1}{\pi a^2}\int_0^a u(x,r,t)\cdot 2\,\pi r dr \tag{14}$$

Using this definition, and inserting this value into the equation of continuity, and integrating the equation across the tube result in the following relations:

$$\pi a\frac{2\partial\bar{u}}{\partial x} + \left\{2\pi r v(x,r,t)\right\}_{r\,=\,0}^{r\,=\,a} = 0$$

The radial velocity at r = 0 must vanish because of symmetry. The radial velocity at r = a is defined by the vibration of the wall and should be calculated from elastic principle. Denote this radial velocity by $v_w(x,t)$, and postpone the calculation for the moment. The last equation yields

$$v_w(x,t) = -\frac{a}{2}\frac{\partial\bar{u}(x,t)}{\partial x} \tag{15}$$

The flowing fluid was assumed to be nonviscous. This permits the use of the equation of motion without the viscous terms

$$\rho\left(\frac{\partial u}{\partial t} + u\frac{\partial u}{\partial x} + v\frac{\partial u}{\partial r}\right) = -\frac{\partial p}{\partial x}$$

$$\rho\left(\frac{\partial v}{\partial t} + u\frac{\partial v}{\partial x} + v\frac{\partial v}{\partial r}\right) = -\frac{\partial p}{\partial r} \tag{16}$$

The approximation of neglecting the viscous terms is a very essential one, as it is implied that the wave travels down the arterial system without any losses. This is definitely wrong, but can be used for the first approximation and should be removed later on. However, Equation 16 is still nonlinear because of the inertia terms. To find the relative magnitude of this nonlinear terms they must be nondimensionalized with the help of characteristic length and velocity, or by choosing characteristic length and time. This can be done by using the speed of propagation of the wave. The speed of propagation, c, which is much larger than the average axial velocity,[6] is given by the product of the wavelength λ, and the frequency f

$$c = f \cdot \lambda \tag{17}$$

The wavelength λ can serve as the characteristic length, while $1/f$ is the characteristic time. The average velocity u will be maintained as the characteristic velocity. Thus the ratio of inertial term to instantaneous acceleration is given by:

$$\frac{u\dfrac{\partial u}{\partial x}}{\dfrac{\partial u}{\partial t}} \sim \frac{\bar{u}\cdot\dfrac{\bar{u}}{\lambda}}{\dfrac{\bar{u}}{1/f}} = \frac{\bar{u}}{f\cdot\lambda} = \frac{\bar{u}}{c}$$

$$\frac{u\dfrac{\partial v}{\partial x}}{\dfrac{\partial v}{\partial t}} \sim \frac{\bar{u}\cdot\dfrac{v^\star}{\lambda}}{\dfrac{v^\star}{1/f}} = \frac{\bar{u}}{c}$$

If the speed of propagation is much higher than the average velocity, as was assumed earlier, these inertial terms can be neglected. It is, however, necessary to evaluate the radial inertia, for which a natural characteristic length is the tube radius, r. The value of v*, the characteristic radial velocity, can be calculated from Equation 15, as the radial wall velocity:

$$v^\star = v_w = -\frac{a}{2}\frac{\partial\bar{u}}{\partial x} \sim \frac{-a\bar{u}}{2\lambda}$$

thus giving:

$$\frac{v\dfrac{\partial u}{\partial r}}{\dfrac{\partial u}{\partial t}} \sim \frac{v^\star\bar{u}/a}{\bar{u}/1_{/f}} \sim -\frac{\bar{u}}{c} \ll 1$$

$$\frac{v\dfrac{\partial u}{\partial r}}{\dfrac{\partial u}{\partial t}} \sim \frac{v^\star\dfrac{v^\star}{a}}{v^\star/1_{/f}} \sim -\frac{\bar{u}}{c} \ll 1$$

It can be concluded that under the previous assumption all the inertial terms are very small compared to instantaneous acceleration, and Equation 16 can be reduced to the following set of differential equations

$$\rho \frac{\partial u}{\partial t} = -\frac{\partial p}{\partial x}$$

$$\rho \frac{\partial v}{\partial t} = -\frac{\partial p}{\partial r} \tag{18}$$

This approximation is appropriate for the cardiovascular system, where the maximum possible value for $\bar{u}/c$ is $0.40/5 = 0.08$, and the average value is about 0.01.

Comparing these two equations, with the use of the characteristic values used in the previous analysis, the ratio is obtained

$$\frac{\frac{\partial p}{\partial r}}{\frac{\partial p}{\partial x}} \sim \frac{a}{\lambda}$$

Since the speed of propagation is very high, and it is known that the frequency is very low (heart beat frequency is about 1 Hz), the wavelength must be very large, and is definitely much higher than the tube radius, so that $\partial p/\partial y$ is much smaller than $\partial p/\partial x$, and if there is no shockwave in the tube, which is a known fact in physiology, it can be assumed in the first equation of Equation 18 that pressure is a function of axial distance and length only.

Integrating the first Equation of 18, with the use of this assumption, leads to the following equation

$$\rho \frac{\partial \bar{u}}{\partial t} = -\frac{\partial p}{\partial x} \tag{19}$$

Since there is a dependence between average axial velocity and wall motion, it is necessary to solve the elasticity equation for tube wall motion under varying internal pressure. The vessel walls are assumed to be Hookian material, namely linear relation between stress and strain

$$\sigma = E \cdot \epsilon \tag{20}$$

and incompressible, so that Poisson's ratio can be taken as 0.5. As the radius expands from a to $a + \eta(x,t)$ the associated strain is

$$\epsilon = \frac{2\pi(a+\eta) - 2\pi a}{2\pi a} = \eta/a$$

The stress per unit length is given by dividing the circumferential tension, T, by the thickness of the tube, h. Thus, given by

$$T = E \cdot h \cdot \frac{\eta(x,t)}{a} \tag{21}$$

This tension must balance the inner pressure and the wall inertia. The balance, as shown in Figure 5, is given by:

tension forces = pressure forces + inertia forces

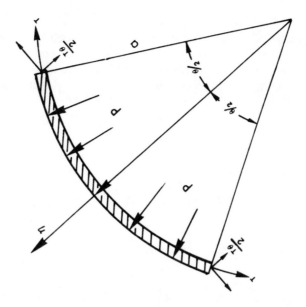

FIGURE 5. Analysis of forces in segment of the arterial wall.

$$\frac{Eh\theta}{a}\eta = a\theta \cdot p - \rho_w(a\theta h)\ddot{\eta} \tag{22}$$

where the term $\sin\theta$ in the left-hand side was replaced by θ. This results in an expression for the pressure as a function of wall motion.

$$p = \frac{Eh}{a^2}\eta + \rho_w h\ddot{\eta} \tag{23}$$

The matching boundary condition requires that at the wall interface both solid and fluid keep in contact, and hence have the same velocity.

$$v_w(x,t) = \dot{\eta}(x,t) \tag{24}$$

This requires simultaneous solution of Equation 23 and Equation 15. However, by neglecting the second term in Equation 23, the inertia term, it is possible to obtain a very simple solution. Using only the first term on the right-hand side of Equation 23 together with Equations 15, 19, and 24, the following wave equations for both the pressure and the average velocity are obtained:

$$\frac{\partial^2 p}{\partial t^2} = c_0^2 \frac{\partial^2 p}{\partial x^2}$$

$$\frac{\partial^2 \bar{u}}{\partial t^2} = c_0^2 \frac{\partial^2 \bar{u}}{\partial x^2} \tag{25}$$

where c_0 is the speed of propagation of both pressure and velocity waves. This value known as the Mones-Korteweg wave speed, is an approximation to the true speed wave, and is given by:

$$c_0 = \left(\frac{Eh}{2a\rho}\right)^{1/2} \tag{26}$$

When Mones introduced this result, that was developed for an elastic rubber tube, he suggested the use of a correction coefficient of 0.90 to 0.95, to match the theory with his experimental results. The reason for this difference is the assumption of non-viscous flow that mean no viscous attenuation of the pressure wave.

The inertial and the viscous terms can be considered analytically if the existence of wave is accepted, and the principle of superposition is used to analyze separately each harmonics of the wave. The relations for the pressure and average velocity are

$$\bar{u}(x,t) = \sum_n A_n e^{i(\alpha_n x - \omega_n t)} = f\left(x - \frac{\omega_n}{\alpha_n} t\right) = f(x - c_n t)$$

$$p(x,t) = \sum_n B_n e^{i(\alpha_n x - \omega_n t)} = g\left(x - \frac{\omega_n}{\alpha_n} t\right) = g(x - c_n t)$$

(27)

where c_n is the assumed speed of propagation. The wave motion is periodical, with a frequency ω, thus

$$\eta = \eta_0 e^{i\omega t}$$

Inserting this relation into Equation 23 results in:

$$p(x,t) = \frac{Eh}{a^2}\eta + \rho_w h(-\omega^2)\eta = \frac{Eh}{a^2}\left(1 - \frac{\omega^2 \rho_w a^2}{E}\right)\eta(x,t) \quad (28)$$

Comparing Equation 28 and the first part of Equation 23 the following speed of propagation is obtained:

$$c = c_0\left[1 - \left(\frac{\omega}{\omega_c}\right)^2\right] \tag{29}$$

where ω_c is the cut-off frequency, given by:

$$\omega_c = \left(\frac{E}{\rho_w a^2}\right)^{1/2}$$

The range of values for this cut-off frequency in the arterial system is always higher than 250 rad/sec (about 40 Hz). It is therefore a very minor correction to the Mones-Korteweg wave speed, (since ω, the frequency of the heart is near 1 Hz), and the use of Mones-Korteweg wave speed as the actual speed of propagation is justified. However, the introduction of viscous term into these equations will result in a complex value for the speed of propagation which means that viscosity introduces damping into the system. This will be considered when the complete set of equations is solved for conditions of pulsatile flow.

As was pointed out by Bergel[1] the actual speed of propagation is larger in the smaller blood vessel than the predicted value given by the Mones-Korteweg equation. This, according to Bergel, is due to the increase in wall thickness, and thus introduces an error by considering the ratio of wall thickness to external rather to the mean radius. In addition there is a change in wall thickness when the pressure is raised, this is due to a nonzero value of the Poisson's ratio. He suggested the following correction for the speed of propagation:

$$c = c_0 \left[\frac{2 - \Upsilon}{2 - 2\Upsilon(1 - \sigma - 2\sigma^2) + \Upsilon^2(1 - \sigma - 2\sigma^2) - 2\sigma^2} \right]^{1/2} \quad (30)$$

where

$$\Upsilon = \frac{h}{R_0}$$

and R_0 is the external radius.

As was pointed out by Bergel, for arteries where $Y = 0.1 - 0.13$ and $\sigma = 0$, the increase in speed of propagation is about 12%. Gow and Taylor[4] modified this expression, by replacing the internal radius of the tube, in Equation 26, with the average radius R_m, described by the external radius as

$$R_m = \frac{2R_0 - h}{2}$$

and by introducing $\sigma = 0.5$ into Equation 29, they obtained the following expression:

$$c = \left[E_{dyn} \frac{h}{2\rho R_M} \right]^{1/2} \cdot \left[\frac{2}{3}(2 - \Upsilon) \right]^{1/2} = \left[\frac{2}{3} E_{dyn} \frac{\Upsilon}{\rho} \right]^{1/2} \quad (31)$$

where E_{dyn} is the dynamic elastic modulus, which is the real part of the complex elastic modulus. They were able to compare the values given by this equation with experimental results. It is, however, acknowledged that all these formulas are not accurate enough, but that the deviations from the real values are less than 10%, which is good enough for the description of the cardiovascular system where changes from one individual to another usually exceed this error.

The comparison of the speed of propagation with experimental results requires the measurement of the elastic modulus as well as the actual thickness of the wall. These two measurements introduce further difficulties in the experimental procedure. To overcome this difficulty it is possible to use the expression for the velocity of sound in air, developed by Newton, and given by:

$$c_0 = \left(\frac{K}{\rho} \right)^{1/2} \quad (32)$$

where K is the bulk elastic modulus describing volume elasticity, and is given by:

$$K = \frac{\delta p}{\left(\frac{\delta v}{v} \right)} \sim \frac{\Delta p}{\frac{\Delta v}{v}} \quad (33)$$

Thus, obtaining the Hill equation for the speed of propagation

$$c_0 = \left[\frac{\Delta p \cdot v}{\rho \cdot \Delta V} \right]^{1/2} = \left[\frac{R \cdot \Delta p}{2\rho \cdot \delta R} \right]^{1/2}$$

The use of this equation eliminates the need to measure the elastic modulus and tube thickness, replacing them with easier measurement of pressure and radial expansion.

E. Wave Reflections — Nonviscous Model

The solution to the pressure-flow relation given by Equation 25, the well-known wave equation, yield the general relations

$$P(x,t) = P_1(x - c_0 t) + P_2(x + c_0 t) + P_0$$

$$\bar{u}(x,t) = u_1(x - c_0 t) + u_2(x + c_0 t) + \bar{u}_0$$

$$(34)$$

These equations describe waves propagating in both directions. The waves the originate by the contraction action of the heart are considered to travel in the positive direction. The waves that travel in the opposite direction are the result of reflections at sites of discontinuities. These discontinuities may be sites of diameter changes, such as branches and bifurcations, or changes in the elastic properties of the wall. The fact that the governing equations are linear allow the separate consideration of the time-dependent components of the wave, while steady flow and average pressure can be ignored during this type of analysis. For the same reason it is possible, for ease of mathematical treatment, to consider each harmonic, when the pulse is written as Fourier series, separately. The actual pressure and average velocity will be given by the vectorial sum of the incident and reflected waves of all of the harmonics.

From Equation 34 and the first of Equation 18 the following relations between pressure and flow are obtained:

$$p(x,t) = p_1(x - c_0 t) + p_2(x + c_0 t)$$

$$\bar{u}(x,t) = \frac{1}{\rho c}[p_1(x - c_0 t) - p_2(x + c_0 t)]$$

$$(35)$$

Two conclusions can be drawn from this equation: 1. The incident and reflected waves at the site of reflection will augment each other; 2. Unlike the reflected pressure, the reflected velocity or flow, is 180° out of phase with the incident wave, and hence, they tend to cancel each other. The actual forward wave is a composite wave composed on the primary incident wave and re-reflections of the backward wave at the heart, and other discontinuities. The backward wave is also a composite wave of reflections at various sites in the circulation system, not only close to the heart but also in the peripheral system.

The flow rate is given by:

$$q(x,t) = \pi a^2 \bar{u}(x,t) = \frac{\pi a^2}{\rho c}[p_1(x - c_0 t) - p_2(x + c_0 t)] \qquad (36)$$

The constant relating pressures and flow rate depends only on tube properties, and is defined by the characteristic impedance,

$$z_0 = \frac{\rho c}{\pi a^2} \qquad (37)$$

The characteristic impedance increases as the tube becomes smaller, and as its elastic modulus increases. Both these phenomena take place in the arterial tree from the aorta toward the periphery. However, the characteristic impedance by itself cannot provide sufficient information to calculate the reflection as a discontinuity. This reflection is the ratio of reflected to incident wave, and as such is a function of time and position. To relate the reflection coefficient to tube properties a definition of longitudinal impedance is necessary. The longitudinal impedance, Z, is defined as the ratio of pressure and flow

$$Z(x,t) = Z_0 \frac{p_1(x - c_0 t) + p_2(x + c_0 t)}{q_1(x - c_0 t) + q_2^{\cdot}(x + c_0 t)}$$

$$= Z_0 \frac{p_1(x - c_0 t) + p_2(x + c_0 t)}{p_1(x - c_0 t) - p_2(x + c_0 t)}$$

$$= Z_0 \frac{1 + \dfrac{p_2(x + c_0 t)}{p_1(x - c_0 t)}}{1 - \dfrac{p_2(x + c_0 t)}{p_1(x - c_0 t)}}$$

and with the definition of the reflection coefficient

$$R_f(x,t) = \frac{p_2(x + c_0 t)}{p_1(x - c_0 t)} \tag{38}$$

the longitudinal impedance is given by

$$Z(x,t) = Z_0 \frac{1 + R_f(x,t)}{1 - R_f(x,t)} \tag{39}$$

Reflection sites are any point where there is a change in the characteristic impedance, either because of a change in diameter, or a change in the elastic properties of the wall. Such changes occur continuously from the ascending aorta down to the capillary bed. It is, however, more convenient to calculate the total resistance of a branch at some determined point rather than calculate reflection from the capillary bed and upstream. This can be done by the use of input impedance, defined as the ratio of pressure and flow at the given point. This results in a complex value, expressing both modulus and phase angle of the impedance. In all the discussion so far the attenuation of the wave is not considered. If the tube is considered as a frictionless tube, and viscosity effect is ignored, the reflected pressure and flow will have the same shape, except with a change in sign. A detailed analysis of the attenuation coefficients is very complex, and will be discussed in the next chapter. It is assumed here, for mathematical ease, that a constant damping factor can be used, thus attenuation depends on the length along which the wave is traveling.

F. Calculation of Reflection Coefficients

To demonstrate the process of finding the reflection coefficient consider two semi-infinite vessel segments joined at the plane $x = 0$. The left vessel, Figure 6, is connected to a pulsatile source. The incident wave $p_1(x,t)$ travels toward the interface, upon reaching the plane $x = 0$ part of the wave is transmitted $p_1(x,t)$, and another portion is reflected as an inverse pressure pulse $p_2(x,t)$, with a flow pulse opposite in sign to the input pulse. Thus upstream of the reflection site the flow and pressure are given by the vectorial sum of forward and backward going waves. It is assumed, because of infinite length, that the transmitted wave suffers no further reflections.

At the interface, $x = 0$, continuity of both pressure and flow must prevail, thus giving:

$$q_1(x - ct) + q_2(x + ct) = q_1'(x - ct)$$

$$p_1(x - ct) + p_2(x + ct) = p_1'(x - ct) \tag{40}$$

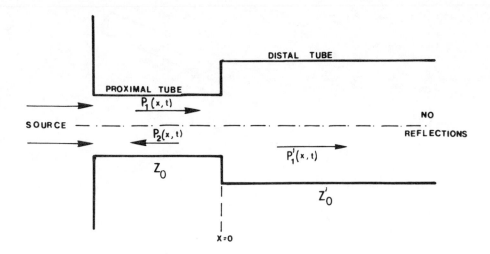

FIGURE 6.   Semiinfinite vessel segment, with expanding interface.

where the speed of propagation c, is replacing the Mones-Korteweg speed of propagation c_0, to make the equation more general. Equation 36 can be used to replace the flow rate with pressures, thus changing the first of Equation 40 to:

$$\frac{1}{z_0} \left[p_1 (x - ct) - p_2 (x + ct) \right] = \frac{1}{z_0'} p_1' (x - ct) \tag{41}$$

Dividing this equation by the second part of Equation 40, and rearranging terms, the following relation is obtained:

$$\frac{z_0}{z_0'} = \frac{1 + R_f(x,t)}{1 - R_f(x,t)} \quad @ \quad x = 0 \tag{42}$$

The ratio between the characteristic impedance of the proximal and distal tubes is, therefore, sufficient to determine the reflection coefficient. Denoting this ratio by λ, gives

$$R_f(0,t) = \frac{1 - \lambda}{1 + \lambda} \tag{43}$$

The value of λ, can be calculated by the use of Equation 37 to give

$$\lambda = \frac{z_0}{z_0'} = \frac{\pi a'^2}{\rho c'} \cdot \frac{\rho c}{\pi a^2} = \frac{c}{c'} \left(\frac{a'}{a} \right)^2 \tag{44}$$

Some conclusions can be obtained from this equation. If there is no change in tube properties, λ is determined by the ratio of cross-sectional area. If there is a sudden change in tube properties without a change in cross-sectional area, the reflection is determined by the square root of the ratio of the elastic modulus.

At the extreme case, when $z_0' \to \infty$, which corresponds to a very small diameter of the distal tube, the value of λ approaches zero, thus giving $R_f (0,t) = 1$. This case, defined as "closed end" result in a complete reflection, without a phase shift. At the other extreme, when the distal tube is very large, thus the characteristic impedance

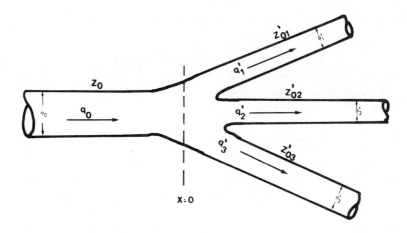

FIGURE 7. General bifurcation.

approaches zero, the value of λ is very large thus giving a reflection coefficient $R_f(0,t)$ = −1. This case defined as "open end" resulting in no amplitude change but a finite phase shift.

According to these findings, the characteristic value λ can be described as the "rigidity" of the discontinuity where the following cases exist:

λ > 1; change from more rigid to less rigid tube (open-end)
λ = 1; matched conditions — no reflections.
λ < 1; change from less rigid to more rigid tube (closed-end)

The case λ = 1, which corresponds to matched conditions can be further explained in an expansion of the previous case, to a case of a general bifurcation, Figure 7. The impedances shown in the figure can be replaced by input impedances to make it a more general case. Ohm's law can be applied to each of the arterial segments

$$q_i = \frac{p}{Z_i} \tag{45}$$

Continuity of flow at the bifurcation gives:

$$q_0 = q_1' + q_2' + \cdots + q_n' = \frac{p_1'}{Z_{0_1}'} + \frac{p_1'}{Z_{0_2}'} + \cdots$$
$$+ \frac{p_1'}{Z_{0_n}'} = \frac{p_1'}{Z_{eq}} \tag{46}$$

where only positive waves are considered in the distal segments. The flow in the proximal tube, q_0, is composed of forward and backward waves, thus giving:

$$\frac{1}{Z_0} \left[p_1(x - ct) - p_2(x + ct) \right] = \frac{1}{Z_{eq}} p_1'(x - ct) \; ; \; @ \; x = 0 \tag{47}$$

and the continuity of pressures:

$$p_1(x - ct) + p_2(x + ct) = p_1'(x - ct) \; ; \; @ \; x = 0 \tag{48}$$

Dividing Equation 47 by Equation 48, and rearranging terms yields

$$\frac{1 - R_f(0,t)}{1 + R_f(0,t)} = \frac{Z_0}{Z_{eq}} = Z_0 \left(\frac{1}{Z'_{0_1}} + \frac{1}{Z'_{0_2}} + \cdots \frac{1}{Z'_{0_n}} \right) = \lambda' \quad (49)$$

which gives the reflection coefficient

$$R_f(0,t) = \frac{1 - \lambda'}{1 + \lambda'} \quad (50)$$

This equation gives the value of the reflection coefficient at any kind of bifurcation. It does neglect the actual flow in the bifurcation, a very complex matter that will be discussed in the next chapter.

If the branching, or bifurcation, involves no change in tube parameters, namely no change of elastic modulus and tube thickness, but only a change in geometry, the reflection is determined by λ', given by:

$$\lambda' = \frac{a_0^{\frac{5}{2}}}{a_1'^{\frac{5}{2}} + a_2'^{\frac{5}{2}} + \cdots a_n'^{\frac{5}{2}}} \quad (51)$$

For the special case, when all distal branches have the same diameter, a_i, this equation reduces to:

$$\lambda' = \frac{1}{n} \left(\frac{a_0}{a_i} \right)^{\frac{5}{2}} \quad (52)$$

It is more convenient to use the total cross-sectional area, rather than the radius of the distal arteries. When this ratio is denoted by K

$$K = \frac{na_i^2}{a_0^2} \quad (53)$$

the value of λ' is given by:

$$\lambda = n^{\frac{1}{4}} \cdot K^{-\frac{5}{4}} \quad (54)$$

In the common case of bifurcation, where $n = 2$, the ratio of cross-sectional area that will provide matched condition of zero reflection can be calculated from Equation 54 by taking $\lambda' = 1$. This will result in an area expansion ratio of 1.15. When the area expands by more than 15%, the value of λ' is smaller than 1, and describes transition into a more rigid tube (closed end). If the area expansion is less than 15% the distal arteries are considered much softer, and represent a finite phase shift with no change in amplitude. In the arterial system the value of area expansion is very close to this calculated value, thus providing very little reflection. However, this changes as the wave is transmitted through smaller and smaller vessels. It should be noted that the vasomotor activity can control this phenomena by changing the cross-sectional area in the periphery.

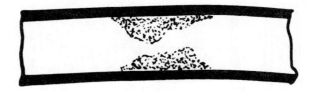

FIGURE 8. Example of stenotic arterial segment, with narrowing of 20% due to plaque formation.

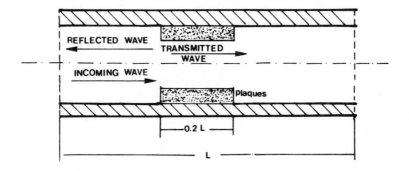

FIGURE 9. Equivalent presentation of stenotic vessel.

As an example, the area expansion ratio at the aorto-iliac junction, is very close to this value in infants. This value declines with age, reaching values of 0.8 to 0.9 at the fourth decade,[2,7] and less than that at the fifth decade.[3,5] This fact not only points to an increase of peripheral rigidity, and toward a behavior of closed end, but also to the fact that the reflection coefficient result is a decrease in the efficiency of the heart pump, since the increased reflection represent an increasing amount of reflected energy that is not used. In addition the increased reflection causes higher pressure above the bifurcation, which might result in an atherosclerosis of the region.

Another example of the use of this technique is the calculation of the pressure buildup in a stenotic artery. Narrowing, or stenosis, of the blood vessel is quite common in the circulatory system. The changes are not only geometric, but also involve a change in elastic properties of the conduit. Consider a case an artery of length L, in which 20% for the length are narrowed due to plaque formation on the wall, Figure 8. For simplicity, the change in propagation speed, which is given by Equation 26 and depends on elastic modulus and tube geometry, is assumed to decrease by one half. This makes the equivalent length of the stenotic segment to double, because the wave travels slower. Thus, the equivalent segment shown in Figure 9 can be considered. The inflow pressure will partially reflect and be partially transmitted at the proximal part of the stenotic area. The reflected part, travels back and re-reflects at the entrance, to pass again through the arterial segment. The transmitted wave, upon reaching the connected impedance, will again split into reflected and transmitted wavelets. To obtain the pressure buildup, all of these wavelets must be added as shown in Figure 10. Assume a regular case where the coefficient of reflection at the stenotic region is 0.6, transmitted coefficient is 0.8. The matched impedance at the outlet result in a reflection coefficient of 0.25, while at the entrance complete reflection (closed end) is assumed. The pressure distribution for this case is compared with two cases. In the first, assume that the waves travel without any reflections and only attenuation, due to energy loss,

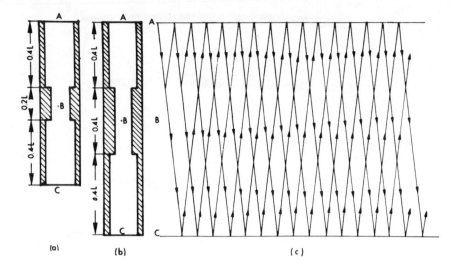

FIGURE 10.   (a) The equivalent stenotic artery. (b) The stenotic region is stretched in order to use uniform speed of wave propagation. (c) The summation of characteristics (incident, transmitted, and reflected waves).

is taking place. In the other case, vasoconstriction of the peripheral circulation is considered and the reflection coefficient is increased to twice this value, namely 0.5.

G. Pressure Buildup in Stenotic Vascular Regions

Narrowing, or stenosis, of blood vessels is quite common in the circulatory system. This narrowing can be caused by various mechanisms, as, for example, fibrin deposition or intravascular plaques. There is a general agreement among researchers, that after deposition of fibrin, or other material, the internal wall of the blood vessel becomes covered with an endothelium layer, and is actually incorporated into the vessel wall. Hence, a stenotic region can be considered as a segment of the artery with a different radius and wall thickness and different elastic properties.

This phenomenon, which is an extremely widespread disease of aging, might lead to myocardial infarction, cerebral thrombosis, and other serious illnesses. Part of the reason for these complications is due to increased systolic pressure observed under stenotic conditions, which causes further development of atherosclerosis. It also alters the shape and peak value of flow and pressure. It is possible to obtain an analytical explanation for the pressure rise and changes in flow rate by the use of the one-dimensional wave characteristics method.

The arterial segment is considered as a straight-walled pipe made of elastic membrane, with changes in diameter or elastic properties permitted only discontinuously at given points. The stenotic area is such a discontinuity. The pressure and flow are assumed to obey the one-dimensional wave equation, discussed before.

The procedure of obtaining an analytical solution is described in a specific example. The length of the stenotic region is taken as 20% of the entire arterial segment length, as shown in Figure 10. The reduction in cross-sectional area is taken as 50%, which corresponds to a 30% reduction in diameter. This will change the thickness of the vessel wall accordingly, and hence will alter the speed of propagation. The speed of propagation is also changed due to the appropriate change in the elastic modulus. It is assumed that the total change of all these parameters is a 50% decrease in the speed of propagation. Thus in the stenotic segment the wave is traveling in half the speed, which doubles the equivalent length of the stenotic area. Thus, it will be assumed that the stenotic length is doubled and the wave transverses the entire arterial segment with the same speed of propagation.

The initial flow condition into the segment is a constant volume flowing into the system during part of the cycle. If these conditions are traced back to the heart, it will mean that the heart is considered as a constant-volume pump. This is achieved by a mechanism of auto-regulation, which actuates intrinsic mechanisms in the brain, kidney, muscles, and other tissues to any persistent rise, or fall, in arterial perfusion pressure and adjusts the peripheral vascular conductance so that the rate of blood flow remains constant. The volume output is assumed to be of the following form:

$$V = Ke^{-at} \sin bt \tag{55}$$

in which a, b, and k are determined in the following way: b is determined by the chosen duration of systole, typical values are from 3π to 5π/sec, which corresponds to 1/5 to 1/3 of the total pulse period; a is chosen to match the known physiological shape, and typical values are from 5 to 15 where t is measured in seconds; k is given by the desired stroke volume, Q which is equal to the integral of Equation 55 over time multiplied by the cross-sectional area A.

$$Q = AK \frac{b}{a^2 + b^2} \tag{56}$$

For the following example the following values are taken:

$$b = 5\pi \frac{1}{sec}, \quad a = 10 \frac{1}{sec}, \quad K = \frac{1}{\rho c}$$

The ratio of tube length to speed of wave propagation is taken as $L/C = 0.01$.

The volume of inflow, given by Equation 56, will generate a pressure wave P, given by a similar relation

$$P = \rho cv = e^{-at} \sin bt \tag{57}$$

that travels down the arterial segment.

The pressure wave travels down the arterial segment. Upon reaching the stenosis, only part of this wave is transmitted through the stenosis, the other part is reflected from the proximal part of the stenosis. The reflected part, P_2, travels back toward the entrance where part is re-reflected to start down the arterial segment again, and the other part is transmitted downstream. The part transmitted through the stenosis, P_1', will again split into reflected, P_1'', and transmitted components upon reaching the exit of the segment and the entrance to the connected impedance, point c in Figure 13. The exact calculation of the reflection coefficients for this case is very complex, and involves the ratio between stenotic length and wavelength. However, when reflection coefficients are considered separately for each discontinuity, the following relations are obtained:

$$\frac{P_2}{P_1} = 0.6 \qquad \frac{P_1'}{P_1} = 0.8 \tag{58}$$

The reflection coefficient at the distal end is determined by the connected impedance and is assumed to be equal to 0.5 for the normal case, half this value, 0.25, for the

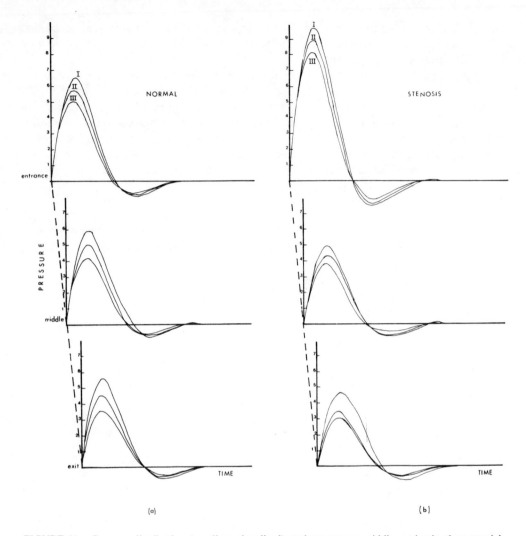

FIGURE 11.   Pressure distribution (nondimensionalized) at the entrance, middle, and exit of an arterial segment for normal (a) and stenotic (b) arteries, for different levels of vasomotor activity.

I.	Vasodilation	$\eta_1 = 0.50;$	$\eta_2 = 0.25;$	$\eta_3 = 0.50$
II.	No vasomotor activity	$\eta_1 = 0.50;$	$\eta_2 = 0.50;$	$\eta_3 = 0.50$
III.	Vasoconstriction	$\eta_1 = 0.50;$	$\eta_2 = 0.75;$	$\eta_3 = 0.50$

(The misalignment of the initial time represents the speed of propagation of the pressure pulse).

case of vasodilatation, and 0.75 for the vasoconstriction case. At the entrance an equal split is assumed, this means that the reflected wave is 50% the incident wave. This results in only a slight back flow toward the larger arteries.

The pressure and flow at any given point is obtained by summing up all the traveling wave, as shown graphically in Figure 10c. The effect of viscosity of the flowing blood and viscoelasticity of the vessel wall is considered by introducing an attenuation of the wave amplitude. This attenuation is taken as exponential, and is chosen in such a way that passing a length equal to five times the length of this given segment the amplitude attenuates to 1% of the incoming wave amplitude.

The results are shown in Figures 11 and 12. For comparison the same arterial segment, without any change in diameter nor in elastic properties, is considered. This case is referred to as the normal case. Figure 11a shows the pressure distribution at the

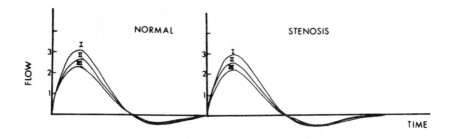

FIGURE 12. Rate of flow (nondimensionalized) in an arterial segment for normal (left) and stenotic (right) arteries for different levels of vasomotor activity (same key as in Figure 11).

entrance, middle of the segment, and at the exit for three cases of normal and under the vasomotor control. If the pressure pulse is considered to be 30 mmHg (120/90), the attenuation for the three cases is given as follows: normal 7 mmHg along the entire segment. For the vasoconstriction the pressure rise is very small, but the attenuation is 11 mmHg for the entire segment, while the attenuation for the vasodilatation case is the lowest, only 4 mmHg. The change in the volume flow of blood, Figure 12, is about 15% for both cases, which is a significant change.

The same results for the stenotic artery, Figure 11b shows that the rise in systolic pressure at the entrance, before the stenosis, is in the order of 15 mmHg, a significant figure that might cause further narrowing of the lumen. Past the stenosis the pressure falls by 7 mmHg in the normal case, and 3 mmHg and 12 mmHg for the vasoconstriction and vasodilatation, respectively. This pressure drop is sometimes sufficient to cause ballooning of the artery distal to the stenotic area. This condition known as poststenotic dilatation causes thrombus formation and further deterioration of the conditions, and worsen the blood circulation. Attentuation for this case is much larger, as can be seen in Figure 11b. This is due to additional energy loss because of the stenotic. However, the change in volumetric blood flow is not as large as the pressure, and blood supply to organ and tissues downstream does not alter significantly, Figure 12b. In this figure only the volume flow rate at the middle is given since they must be equal at any other point in the given segment.

H. The Shape of the Traveling Pressure Pulse Wave

As a consequence of the previous argument it is expected that the branching and discontinuity in impedance in the arterial system will result in the dispersion of the pulse wave. This dispersion of the wave is also due to selective damping of the pulse. It was assumed previously that one attentuation coefficient is sufficient to describe the damping of the pressure pulse. In reality this is not true as the higher harmonics of the pressure wave will undergo a larger attenuation, thus resulting in change of contour in the pressure wave, as it travels downstream.

All the branches and the nonuniformity in the arterial system result in wave reflections. These reflections contribute to a steady rise in systolic peak pressure and a slight decline in the diastolic pressure as the blood moves toward the peripheral circulation. While the contour of the pressure wave gets distorted along its way, significant characteristics, or landmarks, like the dicrotic wave notch will disappear and new hump will be added. Both pressure and velocity have a much sharper upstroke and a much slower descent. There is also a reversal of velocity at the end of systole. In some cases the velocity will reach a short plateau immediately following the peak. However, the contour is continuously changing with time. Because of energy dissipation, and regardless of reflection coefficient, there is no standing waves in the arterial system.

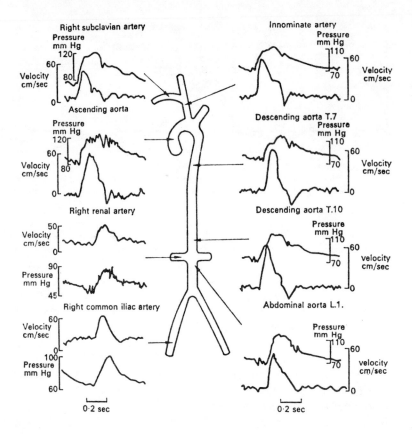

FIGURE 13.   Simultaneous pressure and blood velocity patterns recorded at points in the systemic circulation. (From Mills et al., *Cardiovasc. Res.*, 4, 405, 1970. With permission.)

A typical recording of pressure and velocity patterns in the systemic circulation obtained by Mills et al.[9] from three different patients, as shown in Figure 13. In the second part of their work they changed the segmental requirement for blood and thus the reflection coefficients by taking pressure and velocities during a valsalva maneuver. The results shown in Figure 14 shows that changes in the requirement for blood supply due to a physiological change result in a change in arterial pressure pulse. However, there is not sufficient information to use the pressure pulse for diagnosis of a disease, although many articles appear in the literature describing changes in arterial pulse in health and disease.[10]

I. Composite Waves and Apparent Phase Velocity

As the attenuation of the traveling pulse wave is selective, and different harmonics have different attenuation coefficient, the resulting wave will have a different wavelength. In addition, the pressure at any point is the sum of different waves with different phase angles, that result in a phase angle that changes along the tube. The magnitude of the pressure peak also varies and fluctuates along the tube. To understand the phenomena it is necessary to show the mathematical procedure of dealing with composite waves.

Consider two waves traveling, in opposite direction with different amplitude and different phase angles. The resulting pressure is given by the following relations:

VALSALVA MANOEUVRE

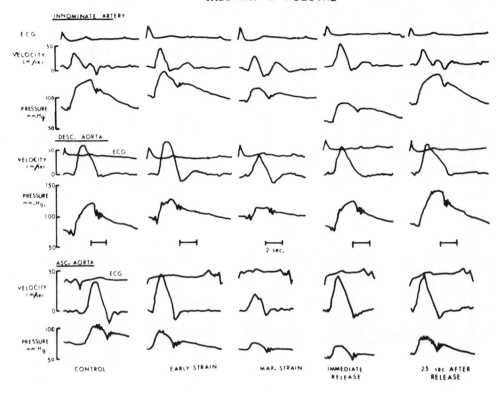

FIGURE 14. Pressure and velocity waveforms and the electrocardiogram recorded during the Valsalva maneuver from the innominate artery and descending aorta at T3 (from same patient) and the ascending aorta (another patient). (From Mills et al., *Cardiovasc. Res.*, 4, 405, 1970. With permission.)

$$P_c = P_1 \cos(\omega t - kx + \phi_1) + P_2 \cos(\omega t + kx + \phi_2)$$
$$= R_e\left[P_1 \, e^{i(\phi_1 - kx)} + P_2 \, e^{i(\phi_2 + kx)} \right] e^{i\omega t} \tag{59}$$
$$= P_c(x) \cdot e^{i\omega t}$$

where $P_c(x)$ is the function that determines both amplitude and pressure. This will change along the tube, and at any given point along the tube the composite pressure will fluctuate in time. This will make it impossible to calculate all the parameters from pressure measurement at a single point. The amplitude of the composite pressure at any given point is given by:

$$P_c(x) = \left[P_1^2 + P_2^2 + 2P_1P_2 \cos(2kx + \phi_2 - \phi_1) \right]^{1/2} \tag{60}$$

If time is kept still and the pressure is measured along the vessel, the result is a pressure wave as shown in Figure 15 where the point of maximum pressure (antinode point) are given

$$2kx + \phi_2 - \phi_1 = 0 ; \quad \pm 2\pi ; \quad \pm 4\pi ; \quad \cdots \tag{61}$$

and the maximum pressure is given by

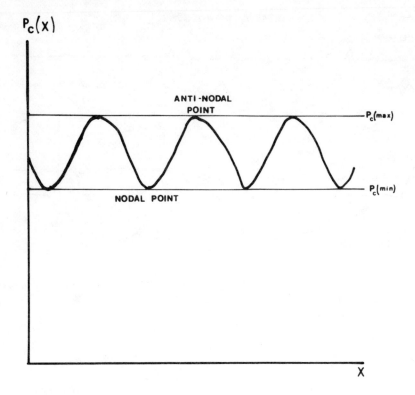

FIGURE 15.   The pressure variation along the blood vessel at a fixed instant in time.

$$P_c(\text{max}) = \left[P_1^{\ 2} + P_2^{\ 2} + 2P_1 P_2 \right]^{1/2} = \mid P_1 + P_2 \mid \qquad (62)$$

The points of minimum pressure (nodal points) are given by:

$$2kx + \phi_2 - \phi_1 = \pm\pi;\ \pm3\pi;\ \pm5\pi;\ \cdots \qquad (63)$$

and the minimum amplitude is given by:

$$P_c(\text{min}) = \left[P_1^{\ 2} + P_2^{\ 2} - 2P_1 P_2 \right]^{1/2} = \mid P_1 - P_2 \mid \qquad (64)$$

From Equations 61 and 63, the distance from node to antinode can be calculated. This distance which is equal to a quarter of a wavelength, as is shown in these two equations:

$$2k(2\Delta x) = 2\pi$$
$$\Delta x = \frac{1}{4}\left(\frac{2\pi}{k}\right) = \frac{\lambda}{4} \qquad (65)$$

If this wavelength is known, a single measurement can give the amplitude of the reflected wave by measuring the pressures at a distance of a quarter wavelength, and summing them with a time delay of a quarter of the pulse duration, as is shown in Figure 16. This will give:

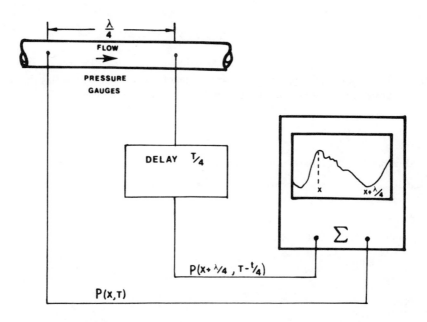

FIGURE 16.   Arrangement for measurements of the reflected wave amplitude.

$$P_c(x,t) + P_c\left(x + \frac{\lambda}{4}; \; t - \frac{T}{4}\right) = 2P_2(x,t) \tag{66}$$

This is true when there is no attenuation present, and with the assumption of standing wave. Thus the ratio of the calculated reflected wave and the calculated incident wave is defined as the standing wave reflection coefficient.

If attenuation is to be considered, the distance which the wave has traveled has to be introduced into the solution, thus changing Equation 66. It will be shown in Chapter 7 that this type of measurement will yield the following relation:

$$P_c(x,t) + P_c\left(x + \frac{\lambda}{4}, \; t - \frac{T}{4}\right) = 2 \cosh \frac{\alpha\lambda}{4} P_2(x,t) \tag{67}$$

where α is the attenuation coefficient.

The average flow and the flow rate which are in phase with each other, has a phase difference with the pressure wave. As the flow rate is given by:

$$q(x,t) = \pi a^2 \, \overline{u}(x,t) = \frac{\pi a^2}{\rho c} \left[P_1 - P_2\right] \tag{68}$$

they will have the amplitude of the pressure wave multiplied by $\pi a^2/\rho c$ but they will be out of phase. The phase difference is equal to a quarter of the period, or a distance of a quarter wavelength. If the ratio between pressure and flow is used to calculate impedance, this phase difference, θ, is very important, since it determines the work done by the system (which is obtained by the product of pressure and rate of flow). The impedance is given by:

$$Z = |Z| e^{i\theta} \tag{69}$$

where Z is calculated by the r.m.s. values of pressure and flow rate. This impedance is a function of position, but not a function of time. If this value of Z is used to determine the apparent phase velocity

$$C = \frac{\pi a^2}{\rho} \left| Z \right| \tag{70}$$

this speed of propagation will also be a function of position. However, it is highly complex to calculate the impedence as it involves a measurement of both pressure and flow. It is convenient to write the pressure wave in the following way:

$$P_c(x,t) = P^*(x) \cos \left[\omega t + \Phi(x) \right] \tag{71}$$

so that the speed of propagation is determined by:

$$C = -\frac{\omega}{\Phi'(x)} \tag{72}$$

For the simple case of no reflection, when the pressure wave is given by:

$$P_c = P_1 \cos (\omega t - kx + \phi_1) \tag{73}$$

will yield

$$C = C_o = -\frac{\omega}{-k} = \sqrt{\frac{Eh}{2a\rho}} \tag{74}$$

The other extreme of closed end with complete reflection

$$P_c = P_1 \left[\cos(\omega t - kx + \phi_1) + \cos(\omega t + kx + \phi_2) \right]$$

$$= P_1 \left[\cos \left(kx + \frac{\phi_2 - \phi_1}{2} \right) \cos \left(\omega t + \frac{\phi_1 + \phi_2}{2} \right) \right] \tag{75}$$

The vibration in this case is all in phase, which corresponds to standing wave, with a constant phase angle. When introduced into Equation 72 it results in an infinite apparent phase velocity. In reality this cannot happen because of attenuation.

In the regular case, the reflection is much smaller than the incident wave, and the composite pressure can be written as:

$$P_c = P_1 \left[\cos (\omega t - kx + \phi_1) + \delta \cos (\omega t + kx + \phi_2) \right] \tag{76}$$

where $\delta \ll 1$.

Asymptotic expansion of this expression for small δ yields:

$$P_c(x,t) = P_1 e^{i\omega t} \left[e^i (\phi_1 - kx + \delta \sin (2kx + \phi_2 - \phi_1)) \right] \tag{77}$$

giving:

$$\Phi(x) = \phi_1 - kx + \delta \sin (2kx + \phi_2 - \phi_1) \tag{78}$$

Inserting the derivative of this last equation into Equation 72 will give:

$$C(x) = \frac{\omega}{k} \frac{1}{1 - 2\delta \cos (2kx + \phi_2 - \phi_1)} \tag{79}$$

Expanding this last term, will give the following approximation for the apparent phase velocity:

$$C = C_0 \left[1 + 2\delta \cos(2kx + \phi_2 - \phi_1) \right]$$ (80)

Hence there are fluctuations along the tube in the apparent phase velocity, about the value of the speed of propagation. The maximum relative deviation is of the order of 2δ, and as such is very small and can be ignored. This is not true in the case of vasoconstriction when the reflection is much bigger, and Equation 80 is not true.

REFERENCES

1. Bergel, D. H., The dynamic elastic properties of the arterial wall, *J. Physiol.*, 156, 458, 1961.
2. Buxton, B. F., Wukasch, D. C., and Cooley, D. A., The dimensions of the Aortollio-Femoral arterial segment, *Aust. NZ J. Surg.*, 42, 204, 1972.
3. Gosling, R. G., Newman, D. L., Bowden, N. L. R., and Twinn, K. W., The area ratio of normal aortic junctions, aortic configuration and pulse-wave reflections, *Br. J. Radiol.*, 44, 850, 1971.
4. Gow, B. S. and Taylor, M. G., Measurement of viscoelastic properties of arteries in the living dog, *Circ. Res.*, 23, 111, 1968.
5. Lallemand, R. C., Gosling, R. G., and Newman, D. L., Role of the bifurcation in atheromatosis of the abdominal aorta, *Surg. Gynecol. Obstet.*, 137, 987, 1973.
6. Luchsinger, P. C., Snell, R. E., Patel, D. J., and Fry, D. L., Instantaneous pressure distribution along the human aorta, *Circ. Res.*, 15, 503, 1964.
7. Malan, E., Noseda, G., and Longo, T., Approach to fluid dynamic problems in reconstuctive vascular surgery, *Surgery*, 66, 334, 1969.
8. McDonald, D., *Blood Flow in Arteries*, Edward Arnold, London, 1960.
9. Mills, C. J., Gabe, J. T., Gault, J. H., Mason, D. T., Ross, J., Braunwald, E., and Shillingford, J. P., Pressure flow relationship and vascular impedance in man, *Cardiovasc. Res.*, 4, 405, 1970.
10. O'Rourke, M. F., The arterial pulse in health and disease, *Am. Heart J.*, 82, 687, 1971.
11. Wiedeman, M. P., Tuma, R. F., and Mayrovitz, H. N., Defining the precapillary sphincter, *Microvasc. Res.*, 12, 71, 1976.
12. Witzig, K., Uber Erzwungene Wellenbewegungen Zaher, Incompressibler Flussigkeiten in elastischen Rohren, Ph.D. Dissertation, University of Bern, Bern, 1914.

Chapter 6

PULSATILE FLOW

A. Experimental Facts on Pressure and Velocity

The intermittent action of the heart and aortic valve, results in a highly pulsatile flow that enters the blood circulation system at the root of the aorta. The existence of a pulsatile flow introduces further complications to the analytical analysis of the pressure-flow relations. Because of this pulsation, the flow cannot be considered as a stable flow except in a relatively small part of the microcirculation. However, this does not mean that the flow is turbulent, although some turbulence might be observed as specific site of the circulation. In spite of the oscillatory nature of the flow it is still, in most instances and in most locations, a laminar flow.

The highly pulsatile nature of the flow that exists in the larger arteries is gradually changing with the branching and tapering of the arterial tree toward the capillary bed. In the small arterioles, prior to entering the capillaries, there are still marked oscillations, that are drastically reduced, and more often disappear distal to the precapillary sphincter. Hence, the flow in the microcirculation is the closest, in the human body, to steady laminar flow. This steady nature of the flow is transferred to the peripheral veins. As the venous flow gets closer to the heart, the suction effect of the right atrium is creating a pulsatile pressure gradient, and hence, a pulsatile flow. In the large veins, closer to the heart, the flow is again highly pulsatile, not only due to the suction of the heart. The respiratory action of the lungs is a major factor in the oscillatory pressure gradient in the venous system, and the determination of venous return. This topic is of utmost importance, and will be discussed in more detail in the appropriate chapter. Another mechanism that contributes to the pulsatile nature of flow in the larger veins is the existence of valves in the smaller veins, which are actually responsible in eliminating back flow in the venous system, and as such are only open with positive pressure gradients.

Typical values of the pressure pulses in the different segment of the circulation are shown in Figure 1. The peaking of systolic pressure in the larger arteries is due to reflection and tapering, as was discussed in the previous chapter. This figure referred to the average pressure, and is different for different harmonics of the pressure pulse.

In determining the flow in the circulatory tree, the pressure is not sufficient and cannot be used as such. The mechanism that determines flow, except vessel impedance, is the pressure gradient. This pressure gradient cannot be calculated, or even predicted, from local pressure measurements. It is dependent on the incident and reflected wave, the relative phase between them, and the site of reflection. However, the average velocity is a linear function of the total cross-sectional area of the blood vessels, and depends on the branching and tapering. An attempt to measure the velocity distribution along the vessel radius, will not reveal a parabolic profile. Near the wall, there will always be a laminae with a very low velocity. This flow, having a very low momentum, will change with a slight change in pressure gradient, and will change direction with the reversal of pressure gradient. The reversal of flow, that starts at the laminae near the wall, gradually diffuses by the mechanism of viscosity toward the axis of the vessel. In some vessels a period of reversed flow can be observed at the end of systole. At these cases, the viscous and inertial terms must be considered equally, and cannot be neglected, as was done in the previous chapter.

B. Pulsatile Flow in Rigid Tubes: Hydrodynamic Equations

A survey of the published literature on the propagation of waves in the arterial system will show a large variation of assumptions on the nature of flow conditions,

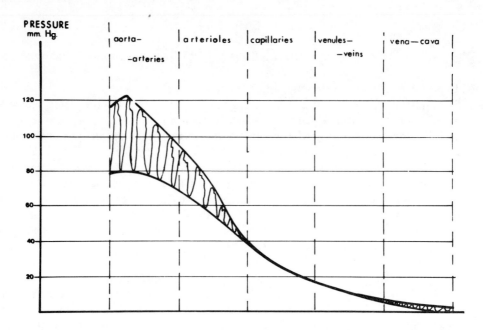

FIGURE 1.   Typical values of the pulsation of pressure in the different segments of the circulation.

fluid properties, and types of vessel walls. The analytical solutions are based on a combination of different assumptions. The most commonly used are summarized in Table 1. The previous chapter discussed the relatively simple case of inviscid fluid, or where viscosity is introduced by a uniform attenuation coefficient. It is, however, expected that viscosity has different effects on different harmonics, and a simple average effect is not accurate enough. The analytical solution for the most general case is too complicated to obtain. It is possible to solve the general case by numerical methods, but this does not permit a study of the contribution of each of these parameters separately.

The most convenient way to examine the relative contribution of the various parameters is to study the flow behavior with certain assumptions, and then to compare the changes in flow distribution as these assumptions are either relaxed or dropped.

Consider first the case of an axisymmetric wave and pulsatile flow with negligible inertia in a rigid tube. The pressure gradient is taken as sinusiodal. This is actually a more general case of periodic pressure gradient, where the pressure gradient is expanded into a Fourier series of the form

$$-\frac{1}{\rho}\frac{dP}{dZ} = \sum_{n=0}^{\infty} a_n \cos nwt = \sum_{n=0}^{\infty} \mathrm{Re}\left(a_n e^{inwt}\right) \tag{1}$$

With the assumptions of circular symmetry, longitudinal velocity only and Newtonian incompressible fluid, the momentum Equation 11 in Chapter 5 has the following form

$$\frac{\partial U}{\partial t} = -\frac{1}{\rho}\frac{\partial P}{\partial Z} + \nu\left(\frac{\partial^2 U}{\partial r^2} + \frac{1}{r}\frac{\partial U}{\partial r}\right) \tag{2}$$

Table 1

Fluid:	Inviscid	
	Incompressible	
	Compressible	
	Viscous $\begin{cases} \text{Newtonian} \\ \text{non-Newtonian} \end{cases}$	
	Multicomponents fluid	
Wall:	Rigid	
	Membrane	
	Infinite thickness	
	Finite thickness	
	Elastic	
	Viscoelastic	
Flow conditions:	Steady state laminar flow $\begin{cases} \text{negligible inertia} \\ \text{nonnegligible inertia} \end{cases}$	
	Pulsatile laminar flow $\begin{cases} \text{negligible inertia} \\ \text{nonnegligible inertia} \end{cases}$	
	Turbulent flow	
Waves:	Axisymmetric	
	Asymmetric	

where U is the longitudinal velocity along the z axis, and with the body forces incorporated into the nonpulsatile component of the pressure gradient. The solution for this component can be obtained separately because of the linearity of Equation 2. This linearity is due to the negligible inertia terms. Inserting the value a_o, from Equation 1 into Equation 2 results in the Poiseuille solution discussed in Chapter 2. For the solution of the other harmonics, a relation of the following form is assumed

$$U(r,t) = f(r) \cdot e^{i\omega_n t} \tag{3}$$

Inserting this equation into Equation 2 and eliminating the time-dependent variables for the nth harmonics results in:

$$\frac{d^2 f}{dr^2} + \frac{1}{r}\frac{df}{dr} - \frac{i\omega_n}{\nu} f = \frac{-a_n}{\nu} \tag{4}$$

Schlichting[24] suggested the following change of variables, to transform this equation into a homogeneous equation

$$S' = r\sqrt{\frac{-i\omega_n}{\nu}} \tag{5}$$

and

$$g(S) = f(r) + \frac{ia_n}{\omega_n} \tag{6}$$

Inserting the new function and new variable, into Equation 4 results in Bessel's equation of the zero order

$$\frac{d^2g}{ds^2} + \frac{1}{s}\frac{dg}{ds} + g = 0 \tag{7}$$

whose solution is given by Bessel functions of the zero order

$$g(S) = c_1 J_0(S) + c_2 Y_0(S) \tag{8}$$

Writing this last equation as a function of radial distance and time gives:

$$U(r,t) = \left[c_1 J_0\left(r\sqrt{\frac{-i\omega_n}{\nu}} \right) + c_2 Y_0\left(r\sqrt{\frac{-i\omega_n}{\nu}} \right) \right] e^{i\omega_n t} \tag{9}$$

This equation must satisfy the boundary condition of no slip at the vessel wall, $r = R$. It also must yield a finite velocity along the tube axis. These boundary conditions result in the following solution:

$$U(r,t) = \operatorname{Re}\left\{ \frac{-ia_n}{\omega_n} e^{i\omega_n t} \left[1 - \frac{J_0\left(r\sqrt{\frac{-i\omega_n}{\nu}} \right)}{J_0\left(R\sqrt{\frac{-i\omega_n}{\nu}} \right)} \right] \right\} \tag{10}$$

Introducing a new nondimensional variable:

$$\alpha^2 = \frac{\omega_n R^2}{\nu} \tag{11}$$

and writing the solution in terms of this variable yield:

$$U(r,t) = \operatorname{Re}\left\{ -\frac{ia_n}{\omega_n} e^{i\omega_n t} \left[1 - \frac{J_0\left(\sqrt{-i}\ \alpha \frac{r}{R} \right)}{J_0\left(\sqrt{-i}\ \alpha \right)} \right] \right\} \tag{12}$$

The new nondimensional is the Reynolds number of the nth harmonics based on frequency. It can be also obtained from the multiplication of the Reynolds number based on velocity, U, and the Strouhal number

$$\alpha^2 = \operatorname{Re} \cdot S_t \tag{13}$$

By expansion of the solution for small and large values of α, it is possible to show that the behavior of the different harmonics is not the same. As α depends on the viscosity of the fluid, it can be concluded that it has a different effect on different harmonics.

Considering the case of small α, Bessel function of first order can be written as:

$$J_0\left(\sqrt{-i}\ \alpha \frac{r}{R} \right) \simeq 1 - \left[\sqrt{-i}\ \alpha \frac{r}{R} \right]^2 = 1 + \frac{i\alpha^2}{4}\frac{r^2}{R^2} \tag{14}$$

so the expansion of the velocity profile for small values of α is given by

$$U(r,t) = \text{Re}\left\{ \frac{-ia_n}{\omega_n} e^{i\omega_n t} \left[1 - \frac{1 + \frac{i\alpha^2 r^2}{4R^2}}{1 + \frac{i\alpha^2 R^2}{4R^2}} \right] \right\}$$

$$= \text{Re}\left\{ \frac{-ia_n}{\omega_n} e^{i\omega_n t} \frac{\frac{i\alpha^2}{4R^2}\left(1 - \frac{r^2}{R^2}\right)}{1 + \frac{i\alpha^2}{4}} \right\} \tag{15}$$

and if $i\alpha2/4$ is neglected compared with 1, the final form of the solution is

$$U(r,t) = \frac{a_n}{4\nu}\left(1 - \frac{r^2}{R^2}\right)\cos\omega_n t \tag{16}$$

This solution corresponds to a Poiseuille flow with a pure parabolic profile, that fluctuates with time. The amplitude for the reversed flow are the same as the forward ones. For the lowest harmonics that correspond to frequency of 8 rad/sec, and blood with viscosity of 4 cp, the largest blood vessel for which the value of α can be taken as sufficiently small, say 0.01, is about 7 μm. It is therefore obvious that this solution is not appropriate for the circulatory system. In the smaller blood vessels, where the value of α is small, the pulsatile nature of the flow has already attenuated. In the larger vessels the expansion for large values of α can be used. For large values of α the expansion of the Bessel function of zero order is given by:

$$J_o(z) \simeq \sqrt{\frac{2}{\P z}} \cdot \frac{e^z}{\sqrt{i}} \tag{17}$$

Inserting this asymptotic expansion into Equation 12 results in the following expression:

$$U(r,t) = \text{Re}\left\{ \frac{-ia_n}{\omega_n} e^{i\omega_n t} \left[1 - \sqrt{\frac{R}{r}} e^{\alpha\left(\frac{r}{R} - 1\right)\left(1 - i\right)\frac{\sqrt{2}}{2}} \right] \right\} \tag{18}$$

The real part of this equation can be calculated to yield:

$$U(r,t) = \frac{a_n}{\omega_n}\left\{ \sin\omega_n t - \sqrt{\frac{R}{r}} e^{-\alpha\frac{\sqrt{2}}{2}\left(1 - \frac{r}{R}\right)} \sin\left[\omega_n t - \frac{\alpha\sqrt{2}}{2}\left(1 - \frac{r}{R}\right)\right] \right\} \tag{19}$$

The result for large α, represented by this equation, has some highly interesting features. The exponential term damps out very rapidly away from the wall. This results in a flow which is independent on radial displacement and viscosity, leaving a boundary layer type flow near the vessel walls. Near the center line of the tube, the fluid

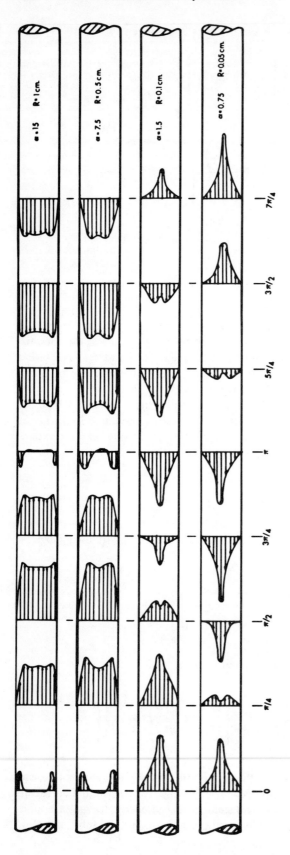

FIGURE 2.   Velocity profiles in a flow generated by sinusoidal pressure for different values of a. The upper curve corresponds to the aorta and the lower curves represent smaller vessels. Note the change in the nature of flow reversal.

behaves like nonviscous fluid for which the flow lags the pressure gradient by half the period. This is true in the aorta, for which the value of α is about 15, as shown in the top part of Figure 2. However, in the smaller vessels the value of α is decreasing, and the nature of the flow is less of a boundary layer type. In the larger vessels there is more of an "annular" type flow, and at no time during the period the flow has a pure parabolic profile. Although this type of flow was observed experimentally in rigid tubes,[22] it does not fit the circulation system because of the elastic nature of the wall. It might represent an approximation to the nature of flow in cases of severe atherosclerosis, when the blood vessels are relatively rigid. In the case of the smaller vessels, the velocity gradients are much larger throughout the tube, thus showing larger dependence on blood viscosity with reversal of flow initiating at the center line of the tube. It should be noted that these results are actually superimposed on a forward Poiseuille-type flow, resulting from the solution of the free term in the Fourier's expansion of the pressure gradient. The relative amplitude of the different harmonics must be considered to determine whether there is an actual "back flow," or if the backward flow of the higher harmonics only reduce the amplitude of the forward Poiseuille flow.

An introduction of the elastic properties of the vessel walls, will permit a displacement of the wall, and hence, must include a radial component of velocity, and a matched fluid-wall boundary conditions.

C. Pulsatile Flow in Elastic Tubes: Hydrodynamic Equations

The assumptions made in the previous chapter are further relaxed by considering the case of an axisymmetric wave and pulsatile flow with negligible inertia in an elastic tube. The pressure gradient is again taken as sinusoidal, assuming that the linerity of the equation enables the use of Fourier's expansion of the pressure gradient, and the use of the law of superposition. The major change is the fact that the fluid must follow the motion of the wall, which is a pulsatile expansion. This necessitates the existence of radial flow component that is much smaller than the longitudinal one, so that the main flow is in the longitudinal direction. This assumption is linked, as was shown before, to another assumption that the tube radius is much smaller than the wavelength. An analytical expression of these assumptions is given by the following relations:

$$\frac{U_{max}}{c} \ll 1$$

$$\frac{|v|}{|u|} \ll 1 \tag{20}$$

$$\frac{a}{\lambda} \ll 1$$

The later assumption was used in Chapter 5 to show that the variations in pressure are a function of longitudinal distance and time only. However, in this analysis the pressure is allowed to vary across the tube. It is a known procedure to assume at this stage that the problem is that of propagating waves at a speed of propagation c and frequency ω. Although these parameters are not known *a priori*, they are to be determined from the solution. The governing equation for the flow are the Navier-Stokes equations, without the inertial term, as described in Chapter 5. Circular symmetry can be inserted into the equation thus giving the following equations:

$$\frac{\partial v}{\partial t} = -\frac{1}{\rho}\frac{\partial p}{\partial r} + \nu\left(\frac{\partial^2 v}{\partial r^2} + \frac{1}{r}\frac{\partial v}{\partial r} - \frac{v}{r^2}\right)$$

$$\frac{\partial u}{\partial t} = -\frac{1}{\rho}\frac{\partial p}{\partial z} + \nu\left(\frac{\partial^2 u}{\partial r^2} + \frac{1}{r}\frac{\partial u}{\partial r}\right)$$

(21)

Together with the equation of continuity

$$\frac{1}{r}\frac{\partial}{\partial r}(rv) + \frac{\partial u}{\partial z} = 0$$

(22)

The solution must match the elasticity equation for the motion of the wall by matching velocity at the interface. However, this matching can be done after obtaining the general solution of the flow field, since Equations 21 and 22 are independent of wall elasticity. The method of solution is presented according to the procedure suggested by Womersley.[31-33] The following parameters are used to nondimensionalize the equations.

$$\alpha^2 = R^2\frac{\omega}{\nu}$$

(23)

$$y = \frac{r}{R}$$

(24)

As the phenomenon is that of a wave propagation, it is appropriate to assume that the variables have the same nature, namely:

$$P(Z, r, t) = P_0(r)e^{i\omega(t - Z/c)}$$

$$u(Z, r, t) = U_0(r)e^{i\omega(t - Z/c)}$$

$$v(Z, r, t) = V_0(r)e^{i\omega(t - Z/c)}$$

(25)

With these assumptions and the equation of continuity, it is possible to show that neglecting the inertia terms is justified.

Inserting these forms into the equation and rearranging the terms the following equations are obtained:

$$\text{radial}\quad \frac{d^2 V_0}{dy^2} + \frac{1}{y}\frac{dV_0}{dy} + \left(i^3\alpha^2 - \frac{1}{y^2}\right)V_0 = \frac{1}{R}\frac{R^2}{\mu}\frac{dP_0}{dy}$$

$$\text{axial}\quad \frac{d^2 U_0}{dy^2} + \frac{1}{y}\frac{dU_0}{dy} + i^3\alpha^2 U_0 = -\frac{i\omega}{c}\frac{R^2}{\mu}P_0$$

(25)

$$\text{continuity}\quad \frac{1}{y}\frac{d}{dy}\left[r_0(y)\right] = \frac{i\omega}{c}RU_0$$

Looking at the equation it is obvious that the homogeneous solution is Bessel function, it is therefore simpler to assume that the pressure is also given by a Bessel function and then try to see if a solution satisfying the equation can be obtained. Thus assuming:

$$P_o(y) = AJ_o(ky) \tag{26}$$

where J_o is a Bessel function of the first kind, order 0, and k is a constant to be determined. A solution based on Equation 26 that satisfies the basic Equation 25 is given by:

$$\text{radial } V_o(y) = c_1 \frac{J_1(i^{3/2}\alpha y)}{J_1(i^{3/2}\alpha)} - \frac{R}{\mu} \frac{Ak}{i^3\alpha^2 - k^2} J_1(ky)$$

$$\text{axial } U_o(y) = c_2 \frac{J_0(i^{3/2}\alpha y)}{J_0(i^{3/2}\alpha)} - i \frac{\omega}{c} \frac{R^2}{\mu} \frac{A}{i^3\alpha^2 - k^2} J_0(ky) \tag{27}$$

These two equations must satisfy the third equation, continuity, and inserting this equation gives the values of k, that is required for this matching

$$k^2 = \left(i \frac{\omega R}{c}\right)^2 = i\left(2\P \frac{R}{\lambda}\right)^2 \tag{28}$$

With the previous assumption it is clear that the value of k in the physiological system is very small (smaller than 0.1). It is therefore appropriate to assume that the Bessel function $J_o(ky)$ and $J_1(ky)$ can be expanded and replaced by

$$J_0(ky) \simeq 1; \quad J_1(ky) \simeq \frac{ky}{2} \tag{29}$$

The matching of solution by the equation of continuity also gives the following relation between the unknown coefficients

$$\frac{c_1}{c_2} = \frac{k}{i^{3/2}\alpha} \tag{30}$$

which reduces the number of coefficients to be determined to two (c_1 and A). The final form of the solution is

$$\text{radial } V_o(y) = i \frac{\omega R}{2c} \left[c_2 \frac{2J_1(i^{3/2}\alpha y)}{\alpha i^{3/2} J_0(i^{3/2}\alpha)} + A \frac{Y}{\rho c} \right] \tag{31}$$

$$\text{axial } U_o(y) = c_2 \frac{J_0(i^{3/2}\alpha y)}{J_0(i^{3/2}\alpha)} + A \frac{1}{\rho c} \tag{32}$$

The determination of the two unknown requires the solution of equations of motion for the blood vessel wall. Only after solving these equations, can the two constants be derived.

D. Pulsatile Flow in Elastic Tubes: Elasticity Equations

The behavior of an elastic tube under distending pressure was discussed in Chapter 4. It is however more convenient to write the equation of elasticity in expressions similar to those obtained for the fluid flow, since this will enable an easier comparison of the type of assumptions used for the description of wall motion. The motion is known to be relatively small, thus allowing the use of linear Hookian relations, described by Equation 21 in Chapter 4. The equations can be written in a different form by using the principal invariant of the stress tensor described by the trace of the stress tensor, θ:

$$\theta = \sigma_{nn} = \sigma_{xx} + \sigma_{yy} + \sigma_{zz} = \text{tr}\sigma \tag{33}$$

From Equation 21 in Chapter 4, the trace of the stress tensor is related to the trace of the strain tensor, ε, by the relation

$$\varepsilon - \varepsilon_{xx} + \varepsilon_{yy} + \varepsilon_{zz} = \text{tr}\varepsilon = \frac{1}{E}(1 - 2\nu)\theta \tag{34}$$

where homogeneity of the wall material was incorporated. The trace of the strain tensor, which is also a principal invariant, is related to the velocity vector by:

$$\varepsilon = \frac{\partial v}{\partial x} + \frac{\partial v}{\partial y} + \frac{\partial v}{\partial z} = \text{div } \vec{v} \tag{35}$$

With these new variables, the normal stress written in matrix form is given by:

$$\begin{pmatrix} \sigma_{xx} \\ \sigma_{yy} \\ \sigma_{zz} \end{pmatrix} = \frac{E}{2(1+\nu)} \begin{pmatrix} 2\dfrac{\partial v_x}{\partial x} & 0 & 0 \\ 0 & 2\dfrac{\partial v_y}{\partial y} & 0 \\ 0 & 0 & 2\dfrac{\partial v_z}{\partial z} \end{pmatrix}$$

$$\tag{36}$$

$$+ \frac{E\nu}{(1+\nu)(1-2\nu)} \begin{pmatrix} \text{div } \vec{v} & 0 & 0 \\ 0 & \text{div } \vec{v} & 0 \\ 0 & 0 & \text{div } \vec{v} \end{pmatrix}$$

and similar expression for the shear stresses:

$$\begin{pmatrix} \sigma_{xy} \\ \sigma_{xz} \\ \sigma_{yz} \end{pmatrix} = \frac{E}{2(1+\nu)} \begin{pmatrix} \dfrac{\partial v_x}{\partial y} + \dfrac{\partial v_y}{\partial x} \\ \dfrac{\partial v_x}{\partial z} + \dfrac{\partial v_z}{\partial x} \\ \dfrac{\partial v_y}{\partial z} + \dfrac{\partial v_z}{\partial y} \end{pmatrix} \tag{37}$$

The last two equations can be combined to give the elastic stress tensor relation given by:

$$\sigma = \frac{E}{2(1+\nu)} \text{ def } \vec{v} + \frac{\nu E}{(1+\nu)(1-2\nu)} \text{ div } \vec{v} \cdot I \tag{38}$$

where def $\vec{v}$ is defined in the following way:

$$
\text{def } \vec{v} = \begin{pmatrix} 2\dfrac{\partial v_x}{\partial x} & \dfrac{\partial v_x}{\partial y} + \dfrac{\partial v_y}{\partial x} & \dfrac{\partial v_x}{\partial z} + \dfrac{\partial v_z}{\partial x} \\[2mm] \dfrac{\partial v_x}{\partial y} + \dfrac{\partial v_y}{\partial x} & 2\dfrac{\partial v_y}{\partial y} & \dfrac{\partial v_y}{\partial z} + \dfrac{\partial v_z}{\partial y} \\[2mm] \dfrac{\partial v_x}{\partial z} + \dfrac{\partial v_z}{\partial x} & \dfrac{\partial v_y}{\partial z} + \dfrac{\partial v_z}{\partial y} & 2\dfrac{\partial v_z}{\partial z} \end{pmatrix} = \nabla \vec{v} + (\nabla \vec{v})^T \tag{39}
$$

where $\nabla \vec{v}$ is a dyadic product of the "del" vector and the velocity vector, and T represents the transpose of this tensor. Equation 38 can be written with the help of Lame's constants G and λ

$$
\sigma = G \text{ def } \vec{v} + \lambda \text{ div } \vec{v} \cdot \sigma \tag{40}
$$

where G is the viscous shearing coefficient or the shear modulus and λ is defined as the bulk coefficient.

The equation of motion for the wall of the blood vessel is given by the general equilibrium condition, Equation 33 in Chapter 4. The external force is obtained by the d'Alambert principle, given by the multiplication of density and the second derivative of the velocity with respect to time. This is the external force per unit volume, thus a body force. Equation 33 in Chapter 4 can be transformed to a tensor equation by:

$$
\rho_w \frac{d^2 v}{\partial t^2} = [\nabla \cdot \sigma] = \text{div } \sigma \tag{41}
$$

where ϱ_w is the density of the wall material.

Inserting the stress-tensor, Equation 40, into the last equation gives:

$$
\rho_w \frac{\partial^2 v}{\partial t^2} = G \text{ div (def } \vec{v}) + \lambda \text{ div (div } \vec{v} \cdot I) =
$$
$$
G \nabla^2 \vec{v} + (G + \lambda) \vec{v} \cdot \text{div } \vec{v} \tag{42}
$$

This is the general equation of motion for elastic walls, in vector notation. For axisymmetric motion of circular cylindrical tube this equation in cylindrical coordinate gives:

$$
\rho_w \frac{\partial^2 v_r}{\partial t^2} = (G + \lambda) \frac{\partial}{\partial r} (\text{div } \vec{v}) +
$$
$$
G \left(\frac{\partial^2 v_r}{\partial r^2} + \frac{1}{r} \frac{\partial v_r}{\partial r} - \frac{v_r}{r^2} + \frac{\partial^2 v_r}{\partial z^2} \right)
$$
$$
\rho_w \frac{\partial^2 v_z}{\partial t^2} = (G + \lambda) \frac{\partial}{\partial z} (\text{div } \vec{v}) +
$$
$$
G \left(\frac{\partial^2 v_z}{\partial r^2} + \frac{1}{r} \frac{\partial v_z}{\partial r} + \frac{\partial^2 v_z}{\partial z^2} \right)
$$
$$\tag{43}$$

This equation has to be solved subjected to boundary conditions on the vessel wall. The internal boundary conditions are those of matched stresses and velocity between fluid and wall. The external boundary conditions are much harder to obtain as they require definitions of tissue motion and interstitial tissue pressure. Because of the later boundary conditions, two possible alternatives are usually carried out. The vessel wall can be considered as infinite in diameter, thus having vanishing stresses and motion, or the other extreme assuming the wall to behave like a membrane. The case of a membrane will be analyzed, however, for easier interpretation and easier boundary conditions, the solution will be obtained using the initial stress-strain relations, and not by expansion of Equation 43, which is another possibility.

As a first approximation consider the case of a thin membrane together with the previous assumptions, especially the assumption of wavelength much longer than tube diameter. In this case, the strains can be considered as constants, and equilibrium conditions are given by a simple balance of the radial and tangential forces, as shown in Figure 3. The balance of forces can be calculated at the midline of the membrane, hence, making it independent of the radial coordinate. This will give:

$$\sigma_{rr} \, R2\Delta\phi = 2\sigma_{\theta\theta} \, h \sin \Delta\phi \simeq 2\sigma_{\theta\theta}h\Delta\phi$$

and from their relations:

$$\sigma_{rr} = \frac{h}{R} \, \sigma_{\theta\theta} \tag{44}$$

The general strain-stress relations, described by Equation 21 in Chapter 4, can be written for the general case of cylindrical coordinates:

$$\epsilon_{rr} = \frac{\sigma_{rr}}{E} - \frac{\nu}{E} \left(\sigma_{\theta\theta} + \sigma_{zz} \right)$$

$$\epsilon_{\theta\theta} = \frac{\sigma_{\theta\theta}}{E} - \frac{\nu}{E} \left(\sigma_{rr} + \sigma_{zz} \right) \tag{45}$$

$$\epsilon_{zz} = \frac{\sigma_{zz}}{E} - \frac{\nu}{E} \left(\sigma_{rr} + \sigma_{\theta\theta} \right)$$

The axial and radial displacements are a function of the longitudinal coordinate and time, but not of the radius, thus:

$$\eta(z,t) = \text{radial displacement of the wall's midline}$$
$$\zeta(z,t) = \text{axial displacement of the wall's midline}$$

With these definitions the strains are given as:

$$\epsilon_{rr} = \frac{\partial n}{\partial r} \, ; \, \epsilon_{\theta\theta} = \frac{n}{r} \, ; \, \epsilon_{zz} = \frac{\partial \zeta}{\partial z} \tag{46}$$

Inserting these values into Equation 45 and elimination of the tangential stress by using Equation 44 (eliminating σ_{zz} by using the last two equations of 45) yield:

$$\sigma_{rr} = \frac{E \dfrac{h}{R}}{1 - \nu^2 - (\nu + \nu^2)\dfrac{h}{R}} \left(\frac{n}{R} + \nu \frac{\partial \zeta}{\partial z} \right) \tag{47}$$

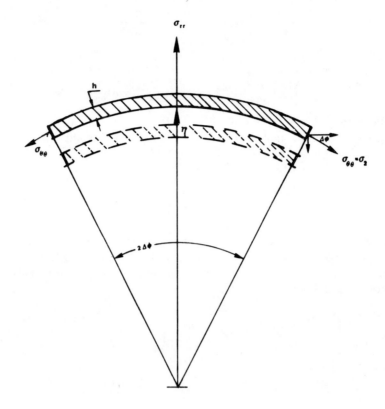

FIGURE 3. Equilibrium condition of radial and tangential forces in a circular segment of the arterial wall.

A fair assumption in the cardiovascular system is the small value of h/R in comparison to unit. Normal range for this value are 0.16 and lower. This assumption reduces Equation 47 to the following relation:

$$\sigma_{rr} = \frac{E \frac{h}{R}}{1 - \nu^2} \left(\frac{\eta}{R} + \nu \frac{\partial \zeta}{\partial z} \right)$$ (48)

Again, using Equation 44 and the relation obtained for σ_{rr}, it is possible to rewrite the last equation in 45 to give the axial stress:

$$\sigma_{zz} = \frac{E}{1 - \nu^2} \left[\left(\nu + \nu \frac{h}{R} \right) \frac{\eta}{R} + \left(1 + \nu^2 \frac{h}{R} \right) \frac{\partial \zeta}{\partial z} \right]$$ (49)

which for small values of h/R is reduced to:

$$\sigma_{zz} = \frac{E}{1 - \nu^2} \left(\nu \frac{\eta}{R} + \frac{\partial \zeta}{\partial z} \right)$$ (50)

To obtain the equation of motion for the vessel wall these stresses must be combined with the accelerative forces and the stresses exerted by the fluid and given by the following relations:

$$\sigma_{rr} = P(z,t) - 2\mu \left(\frac{\partial v}{\partial r}\right)_{wall}$$

$$\sigma_{rz} = \mu \left(\frac{\partial u}{\partial r} + \frac{\partial v}{\partial z}\right)_{wall}$$

(51)

By the assumptions used in obtaining the flow conditions, or by using the solution and neglecting terms of smaller order, these relations can be simplified to give:

$$\sigma_{rr} = P(z,t)$$

$$\sigma_{rz} = \mu \left(\frac{\partial u}{\partial r}\right)_{wall}$$

(52)

Combining all these forces has to result in equilibrium. For the axial force component, the difference between the normal stress in the axial direction is reduced in the limit to the derivative of the normal stress along the axial direction. This will result in the following equations of motion:

$$radial \quad \rho_w h \frac{\partial^2 \eta}{\partial t^2} = P(z,t) - \frac{E \frac{h}{R}}{1-\nu^2} \left(\frac{\eta}{R} + \nu \frac{\partial \zeta}{\partial z}\right)$$

$$axial \quad \rho_w h \frac{\partial^2 \zeta}{\partial t^2} = \frac{E h}{1-\nu^2} \left(\frac{\nu}{R} \frac{\partial \eta}{\partial z} + \frac{\partial^2 \zeta}{\partial z^2}\right) - \mu \left(\frac{\partial u}{\partial r}\right)_{wall}$$

(53)

The solution can be expanded to include the inertia of the surrounding tissue that the wall has to push in its expansion. This is done by replacing the wall thickness by a larger value, H, that includes the tissue. If the density of the tissue is ϱ_t, and the equivalent tissue thickness is h_1, resulting in an annular R_1, the equivalent thickness of the tube is

$$H = h + \frac{\rho_t R_1}{\rho_w R}$$

(54)

Another phenomenon that the equation of motion does not include is the "tethering" of the vessel wall, which results in an additional force exerted by the surrounding tissue. This force is a resistance to motion in the axial direction. Womersley[31,32] accounted for this force by adding another term, proportional to the axial displacement of the midline, to the right-hand side of Equation 53. This force is due to an external elastic constraint and can be represented by a uniform spring constant K, which is determined per unit area of the inner wall. When divided by ϱH, this constant, defined as m^2 by Womersley, was shown to be undamped natural frequency in the longitudinal direction of a wall element. Introducing this term into the axial equation results in the following form:

$$axial \quad \rho_w H \frac{\partial^2 \zeta}{\partial t^2} = \frac{EH}{1-\nu^2} \left(\frac{\nu}{R} \frac{\partial \eta}{\partial z} + \frac{\partial^2 \zeta}{\partial z^2}\right) - \mu \left(\frac{\partial u}{\partial r}\right)_{wall} - K\zeta$$

(55)

The boundary conditions for the elastic and hydrodynamic equations for the velocities are matched velocity at the interface, namely:

$$u(z, R, t) = \frac{\partial \zeta}{\partial t} (Z, t)$$

$$v(z, R, t) = \frac{\partial \eta}{\partial t} (z, t)$$

(56)

As the phenomenon was assumed to be that of a wave propagated along the tube, and agreement with the assumptions leading to Equation 25, the velocity of the wall can be taken as:

$$\eta (z, t) = \eta_0 e^{i\omega \left(t - \frac{z}{c}\right)}$$

$$\zeta (z, t) = \zeta_0 e^{i\omega \left(t - \frac{z}{c}\right)}$$

(57)

where η_0 and ζ_0 are constants to be determined by inserting these values into the equations and boundary conditions.

E. Solutions to Pulsatile Flow in Elastic Tubes

The solution to this problem can be obtained for three different cases: elastic tube, viscoelastic tube, and elastic thick wall surrounded by the tissue. And indeed different solutions appear in the literature. However, the solution to this problem is usually referred to as Womersley's solution, following his elaborate work published in 1955 and 1957; although the first published work that presented a solution to this problem appeared 30 years earlier. Witzig[30] presented the first solution to the problem, but his work that was published in German remained unknown until the early 1950s, when additional solutions were suggested. Most of these solutions, like Aperia,[1] Iberall,[8] Lambossy,[11] and Morgan and Kiely[17] offered general mathematical solutions with various assumptions but mainly related to the case of rigid tubes. Womersley's solution is based on the previous analysis, with Equations 31, 32, 53, and 55 as the governing equations.

For the case of a rigid tube the boundary conditions are reduced to $U_0 (1) = 0$, inserting this value in Equation 32 gives the solution for a rigid tube:

$$U_0 (y) = \frac{A}{\rho c} \left[1 - \frac{J_0 (i^{3/2} \alpha y)}{J_0 (i^{3/2} \alpha)} \right]$$

(58)

Womersley obtained the same solution by assuming a pressure gradient of the form:

$$\frac{\partial P}{\partial z} = A^* e^{iwt}$$

instead of the Bessel function considered in Equation 26, where A^* is a complex constant. An example for a particular set of parameters was described by McDonald[13] and is shown in Figure 4. The velocity profiles are similar to those obtained in Section B, and shown in Figure 2. It is evident from these profiles that the laminae near the wall have the highest velocity gradient, and thus having the highest shear stresses. The flow is gradually moving from the external laminae toward the center of the tube.

The cases for elastic and viscoelastic materials for the blood vessel walls can be combined into the same solution, except in the later case the elastic modulus and the Poisson's ratio are complex functions.

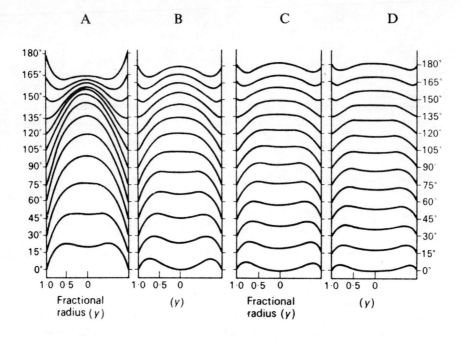

FIGURE 4.   Velocity profiles of flow resulting from sinusoidal pressure, for different harmonics, shown for half a cycle at intervals of 15°.

For the case of pulsatile flow in elastic tubes, the assumption of Equation 56 must coincide with Equations 31 and 32 to yield the boundary conditions given by Equation 56. It also must satisfy the axial and radial equations of motion given by Equations 55 and 53, respectively. If this procedure is carried out, four homogeneous algebraic equations are obtained for four unknown constants $(A, c_1, \eta_o, \zeta_o)$.

$$c_2 \qquad + \frac{A}{\rho c} \qquad\qquad - iw\zeta_o \qquad\qquad = 0$$

$$c_2 \left(\frac{i\omega R}{2c} F_{10} \right) + A \frac{i\omega R}{2\rho c^2} - i\omega \eta_o \qquad\qquad = 0$$

$$\qquad + A \qquad + \eta_o \left(\rho_w H\omega^2 - \frac{BH}{R^2} \right) + \zeta_o \left(\frac{r\omega BH\nu}{CR^2} \right) \qquad = 0$$

$$c_2 \left(-\frac{i\omega\rho R}{2} F_{10} \right) \qquad + \eta_o \left(\frac{-i\omega}{c} \frac{BH\nu}{R} \right) + \zeta_o \left(\rho_w H\omega^2 - \frac{\omega^2}{c^2} BH - K \right) = 0$$

$$(59)$$

where F_{10} is parameter defined by Womersley as:

$$F_{10} = \frac{2J_1 (i^{3/2}\alpha)}{\alpha i^{3/2} J_0 (i^{3/2}\alpha)} \qquad\qquad (60)$$

and B is defined as:

$$B = \frac{E}{1 - \nu^2} \qquad\qquad (61)$$

For the solution to be nontrivial, the coefficient determinant of this set of equations must equal zero. This results in an equation that determines the speed of propagation.

$$
\begin{vmatrix}
1 & \dfrac{1}{\rho c} & 0 & -i\omega \\[2ex]
\dfrac{i\omega R}{2c} F_{10} & \dfrac{i\omega R}{2\rho c^2} & -i\omega & 0 \\[2ex]
0 & 1 & \rho_w H \omega^2 - \dfrac{BH}{R^2} & \dfrac{i\omega BH\nu}{cR} \\[2ex]
\dfrac{-i\omega\rho R}{2} F_{10} & 0 & \dfrac{-i\omega BH\nu}{Rc} & \rho_w H \omega^2 - \dfrac{\omega^2}{c^2} BH - K
\end{vmatrix} = 0
\tag{62}
$$

This equation can be reduced by certain algebraic manipulations to the following expression

$$
\begin{vmatrix}
\dfrac{R}{2\rho c^2}(1 - F_{10}) & 0 & \dfrac{R}{2c} F_{10} \\[2ex]
1 & \dfrac{BH}{R^2} - \rho_w H\omega^2 & \dfrac{BH\nu}{Rc} \\[2ex]
\dfrac{R}{2c^2} & \dfrac{BH\nu}{Rc} + \rho & \dfrac{k}{\omega^2} + \dfrac{BH}{c^2} - \rho_w H
\end{vmatrix} = 0
\tag{63}
$$

Womersley defined new additional parameters to bring this equation to an approximated explicit solution for the speed of propagation c. However, with all of his definitions and approximations it still remains a procedure that requires solutions of few implicit equations. The reason he used this procedure is the difficulty in solving numerical problems. He actually used the computers at the Aiken Computer Center at Harvard University to establish tables for some of the parameters and the solutions. With the availability of computers this equation can be solved directly for the calculation of c for any given set of parameters. It is, however, of importance to discuss the physical meaning of this speed of propagation. This can be done for the simple case of large values of K.

For this case the a_{33} term of the determinant is the dominant term, and hence for this case the approximated solution to the equation is:

$$
\begin{vmatrix}
\dfrac{R}{2\rho c^2}(1 - F_{10}) & -1 \\[2ex]
1 & \dfrac{BH}{R^2} - \rho_w H\omega^2
\end{vmatrix} = 0
\tag{64}
$$

which gives:

$$
c^2 = \frac{BH}{2R\rho}(1 - F_{10})\left(1 - \frac{\rho_w R^2 \omega^2}{B}\right) \simeq \frac{BH}{2R\rho}(1 - F_{10})
\tag{65}
$$

The term, BH/2R is related to the previously defined ideal speed of propagation. Thus the last expression can be changed to:

$$c = c_o \left[\frac{1 - F_{10}}{1 - \nu^2} \right]^{\frac{1}{2}} \tag{66}$$

This is a complex function, and according to Womersely's suggestion, can be separated into real and imaginary parts by the following definition:

$$\frac{c_o}{c} = x - iY \tag{67}$$

The phase velocity is given by C_o/x and the attenuation constant of the propagated wave is given by $2 \P Y/c_o$. From the form of the pressure and velocity waves, Equation 25, it follows that the wave travels at a velocity c_o/x, and the amplitude is being reduced at the ratio of exp $-2 \P y/x$ for each wavelength of travel. Womersley[34] tabulated the values of the phase velocity and the attenuation for a large spectrum of values. With the knowledge of the complex speed of propagation c, all the unknowns in Equations 59 can be evaluated in terms of the pressure gradient's amplitude A. Thus given the solution as a function of the pressure gradient.

An example of the ratio of the true phase velocity and the ideal speed of propagation is shown in Figure 5, for values of α up to 10, and different value of the parameter K. Figure 6 describes the attenuation coefficient for the same values of the parameters. It is evident from these figures that for the physiological range, $\alpha = 3$, the dependent on the parameter K is not so significant, and the true phase velocity is nearly 90% of the original. This value corresponds to the correction coefficient suggested by Mones[16] to fit his theory to his experiments. Also shown in the figures is that after traveling one wavelength the wave amplitude is decreased to nearly 15% of the original pulse. However, one wavelength is much larger than any single segment with no branches in the circulatory tree. The results also correspond to the fact mentioned earlier that the higher harmonies are attenuated at a higher rate, and are therefore damped out first, thus changing the shape of the pulse wave as it travels downstream. This explains the reason for the disappearance of the dicrotic notch at the smaller blood vessels.

The Young modulus and the Poisson ratio can be considered in the previous analysis as complex numbers. This can represent the case of viscoelastic wall, with the real part describing the elastic parameters, and the imaginary part describing the viscous parameters. According to Womersley the complex parameters can be written as:

$$E_c = E (1 + i\omega\Delta E)$$
$$\nu_c = \nu (1 + i\omega\Delta\nu) \tag{68}$$

with the $i\omega$ representing first order derivatives with respect to time. Hence, the viscoelasticity of the vessel wall is considered as a first order system. When introduced into Equation 65, it gives the following relations for the speed of propagation:

$$c = \left[\frac{E_c H}{2R (1 - \nu_c^2)} (1 - F_{10}) \right]^{\frac{1}{2}} \tag{69}$$

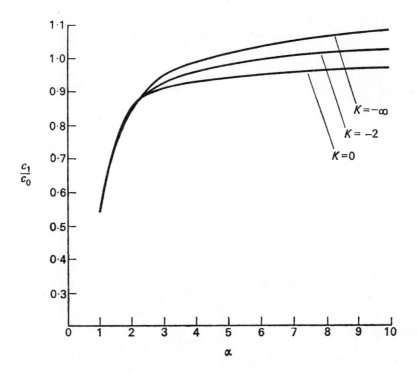

FIGURE 5. Variation of phase velocity of the wave as a function of a, for viscous fluid in a perfectly elastic tube. (From Womersley, J. R., *Phys. Med. Biol.*, 2, 178, 1957. With permission.)

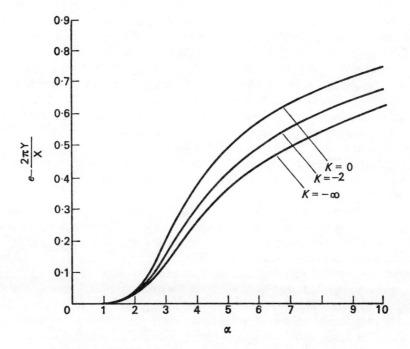

FIGURE 6. Attentuation of the traveling wave as a function of a, for viscous flow in a perfectly elastic tube. (From Womersley, J. R., *Phys. Med. Biol.*, 2, 178, 1957. With permission.)

which after expansion is given by:

$$c = \left[\frac{E\,H}{2R\rho(1-\nu^2)}(1-F_{10}) \right]^{1/2} \frac{1}{1-i\omega W}$$

(70)

$$= \frac{c_0}{(x-iY)(1-i\omega W)}$$

where

$$W = \frac{\Delta E}{2} + \frac{\Delta \nu}{3}$$

(71)

This changes the phase velocity to:

$$c_1 = \frac{c_0}{x}\ \frac{1}{\left(1-\frac{Y}{x}\omega W\right)}$$

(72)

and the attenuation coefficient to:

$$\exp\left[-2\P\ \frac{Y}{x}\ \frac{1+\frac{x}{Y}\omega W}{1-\frac{Y}{x}\omega W} \right]$$

(73)

Since the value of Y/x is small in most arteries of the human circulation system, it follows that viscoelasticity has a minimal effect on the phase velocity, Equation 72. However, the attenuation coefficient, Equation 73, can be several times that of elastic tubes, thus diminishing the pulsatile nature of the flow much faster.

The value of ωW in the human circulation was found to be in the order of 0.1 by Bergel[3] and slightly higher by McDonald and Gessner.[14] This value changes very little with frequency. Taylor[28] determined these parameters experimentally in a rubber tube. His results are shown in Figures 7 and 8 together with the theoretical prediction. There is a very good agreement for the speed of propagation which depends very little on viscoelasticity, and as expected a large deviation from the elastic vessel for the attenuation coefficient. The different numbers in Figure 8 refer to different fluids with different viscosity. Taylor related his findings to an electrical analogue, a topic which is to be considered later.

In an attempt to study the displacement of the tissues due to the pulsatile motion of the vessel, for the possibility of monitoring vessel motion from measurement on the skin, Dinnar[5] solved this problem by considering the wall as a finite thickness tube, surrounded by tissues. Both vessel wall and surrounding tissues were considered as viscoelastic. This necessitated the solution of the complete elastic equation for the tube, solved simultaneously with the elastic equation for tissue motion, with matched boundary conditions at both fluid-wall and wall-tissue interfaces. An added boundary condition is the radiation condition of waves in the out-going direction only and diminishing stresses. The result shows very little effect on the phase velocity and a very large influence on the attentuation coefficient. The results show that increase in the solid elasticity of the tissue will increase slightly the phase velocity and will decrease the attenuation coefficient, as shown in Figures 9 and 10. An increase in the viscous parameter of the tissue will increase both phase velocity and attenuation coefficient.

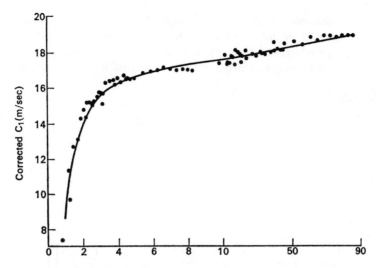

FIGURE 7. Corrected phase velocity, as a function of a. Solid line represents Womersley's solution and the dots represent experimental findings. (From Taylor, M. G., *Phys. Med. Biol.*, 4, 63, 1959. With permission.)

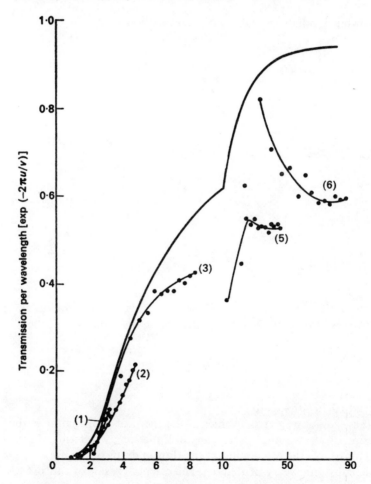

FIGURE 8. Transmission per wavelength as a function of a, for the same experiments used in Figure 7. The solid line represents Womersley's solution, and the experiments are grouped together for different viscosity. (From Taylor, M. G., *Phys. Med. Biol.*, 4, 63, 1959. With permission.)

These results explain why pulsating flow can be detected in arteries that, according to Womersley's solution, should have only the steady component. Similar results were predicted for large arteries by Mirsky[15] who used orthotropic elastic tube, and by Atabek[2] who used a mechanical model consisting of an additional mass, a dashpot, and a spring.

The analytical solution is much more complicated than the previous one since it involves Bessel functions of both kinds in the two added regions of vessel wall and tissue. The results are given by the following expression:

$$\frac{c_0}{c} = x - iY = \left[3W \frac{1-S}{2S} \right]^{\frac{1}{2}} \tag{74}$$

where W is the solution of the following equation:

$$\left(\frac{ZS^2}{P} - 1 \right) \left[Q + f(W) + f(W-1) \right] - R \left[f(W) - f\left(W - \frac{1}{g}\right) \right]$$

$$= -\frac{iR}{g} - \frac{ZS^2}{P} \frac{2 \ln S}{\P} \tag{75}$$

The following nondimensional groups and function were used:

$$Z = \frac{g-1}{g+1}$$

$$S = \frac{R_2}{R_1}$$

$$P = 1 - \frac{1 - F_{10}}{F_{10}} \left[(1 - ZS^2) + W(1 + ZS^2) \right]$$

$$Q = B_2 + i + \frac{1}{\P} \ln \left(\frac{\alpha \mu \omega}{4 \mu_w S^2} \right) \tag{76}$$

$$R = \frac{1}{S^2} - 1$$

$$f(x) = \frac{1}{\P} x \ln x$$

g is the ratio of tissue viscosity to wall viscosity, R_2 is the outer radius and R_1 the inner radius of the vessel wall and B_2 is the coefficient in the expansion of the Bessel function

$$Y_0(x) \simeq \frac{2}{\P} \ln \frac{x}{2} + B_2$$

and is equal to $0.36746 + o(10^{-6})$.

All of these solutions give the values of the speed of propagation c, thus permitting an evaluation of all the other parameters in Equation 59 in terms of the pressure gradient A. This enable the calculation of the flow in terms of the pressure gradient. This is a very lengthy and weary procedure. The essential result of this process can be obtained from the results of the elastic vessel case. If this process is carried out and the result is integrated across the lumen, the following expression for the instantaneous average blood velocity is obtained:

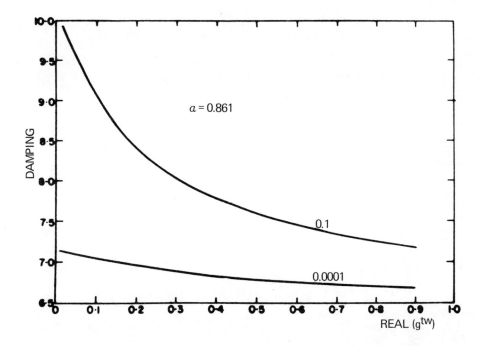

FIGURE 9. Damping of wave amplitude over one wavelength as a function of the real part of the ratio of tissue and wall viscosity. The value of a is 0.861.

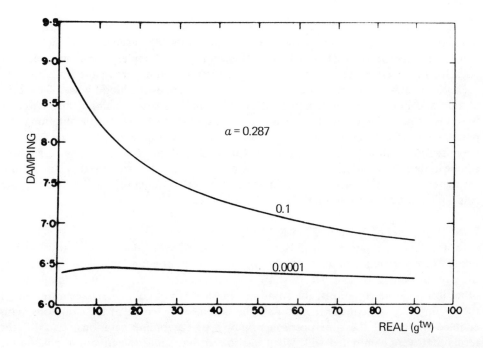

FIGURE 10. Damping of wave amplitude over one wavelength as a function of the real part of the ratio between tissue and wall viscosity. The value of a is 0.287.

$$\bar{u} = \frac{A}{\rho c} \left(1 + \psi\, F_{10}\right) e^{i\omega \left(t - \frac{z}{c}\right)} \tag{77}$$

where ψ is a function of the system's parameters only, given by:

$$\psi = \frac{1}{F_{10} - 2\nu} \left(\frac{2}{x} + 2\nu - 1\right) \tag{78}$$

x is given by the solution to:

$$(1 - \nu^2)x = G \pm \sqrt{G^2 - H'(1 - \nu^2)} \tag{79}$$

in which

$$G = \frac{\frac{5}{4} - \nu}{1 - F_{10}} + k' + \nu - \frac{1}{4}$$

$$H' = \frac{1 + 2k'}{1 - F_{10}} - 1 \tag{80}$$

$$k' = \frac{H\rho_w}{R\rho} \left(1 - \frac{k}{\rho Hw^2}\right)$$

The main conclusion that can be obtained from this result is that the average flow is a sinusoidal one, in which the amplitude depends on the parameters of the system. Since the value of $A/\rho c\,(1 + \psi F_{10})$ in Equation 77 is complex, the amplitude and phase of this average velocity depends on the viscous parameters of the flow, the viscoelastic parameters of the vessel wall and the geometry of the blood vessel. The amplitude and phase are different for different harmonics thus causing a distortion of the pulse shape. However, this result is too complex to be useful in obtaining the parameters from the measurement of this distortion, especially in light of the fact that they assume unidirectional wave propagation and neglect reflections. The reflections can be added to the solution because of the assumption of linearity used in eliminating the inertia terms, this, however, complicates further the already complex form of the solution making it much harder to be of clinical value.

F. Nonlinearities of Pulsatile Flow in Elastic Tubes

In writing the equations for pulsatile flow in elastic tubes there were many assumptions. They were made in order to obtain a soluble set of equations. Although each of the assumptions was justified by showing that a specific term is much smaller than other terms in the equations, the solution obtained is not completely accurate. All of the assumptions were made to eliminate the nonlinearity nature of the equations. This enabled the use of the superposition principle of combining solutions. Each of the terms that were eliminated will, when introduced back into the equation, change the nonlinear nature of the equation. Thus, preventing the use of Fourier expansions of the pressure gradient and the consideration of each harmonics separately. The phenomena that were dropped out of the previous solution, and that will cause the equations to be nonlinear are

1.   The nonlinear connective acceleration terms in the Navier-Stokes equations

2. The large deformation and finite thickness of the arterial wall
3. The geometric and constitive nonlinearities of the blood vessels
4. The viscoelastic nature of the flowing blood
5. The distance along the arterial segment
6. The effect of side branching and division of the blood vessel

Various attempts to include one or several of these factors were published in the literature.

The solution to the nonlinear equations, obtained when these terms are included in the equations, can be obtained in one of three methods. The methods which are relatively the simplest are the methods of characteristics. They are similar to the wave characteristics discussed earlier, except for additional terms. The assumption of one-dimensional flow must still be included, and the solution is obtained by integration of the characteristics. Lambert[10] used this method to include the nonlinear convective terms of the equation of motion and the nonlinearities of the stress-strain curve of human tissue. He found that the effects of the nonlinearities can be very significant and might form a shock wave within the blood vessel. However, his numerical results are not accurate because as was pointed out by Olsen and Shapiro,[21] "He assumed the flow speed to be many times the wave speed, instead of vice versa." They used the correction for long speed wave. However, the boundary conditions that they used assume no pulsation at the downstream section of the arterial segment. In the human body there is no single arterial segment that is long enough to damp out the pulsatile nature of the flow. But even with this extreme attenuation they showed that the effect of the nonlinearities is relatively small. Additional work using the integration of the nonlinear characteristic equations were published by Streeter et al.,[26,27] Iberall,[9] and Skalak and Stathis[25] that included these same parameters and in addition the effect of side branching and division of blood vessels.

When the solution for the three-dimensional flow is desired, the method of characteristics is no more adequate. One of two methods can be used. If the nonlinearities are considered *a priori* to be very small the perturbation method can be used. Without this assumption a numerical solution, most usually by the finite difference method, is the only other possibility.

As an example for the perturbation method the following papers can supply the information: Uchida,[29] Morgan and Ferrante,[18] and Olsen and Shapiro.[21] Ling and Atabek[12] presented a numerical integration of the nonlinear equations using the method of finite differences, together with the consideration for large deformation of the vessel wall.

For the cases where the flowing blood is taken as a viscoelastic material a complex viscosity can be taken. This can be done for each of the procedures described so far. This will no doubt change the amplitude and phase of the various quantities, but will not change the mathematical procedure.

G. Stability of Pulsatile Flow

In a discussion of stability in a case of pulsatile flow, it is essential to define very clearly what are the conditions for a transition from a stable to unstable situation.

The flow in the larger arteries is highly pulsatile, while in the smaller blood vessel most of these pulsatile elements have been diminished, and the flow can be considered as practically steady. Although in the larger vessels the flow can also be stable, despite the fact that there is pulsation. In the capillaries the flow is steady, and on the route toward the heart the flow in the veins becomes pulsatile again, because of the pumping action of the heart and because of pressure variations in the thoracic cavity due to respiration.

It is therefore necessary to discuss separately the different size of vessels and to define instability for each one of them. When calculating the Reynolds number in each of these vessels the value is much smaller than the critical value for transition to turbulence. However, the presence of branching and other fluid wall interaction results in instability of flow. This instability has to be distinguished from turbulence. The term turbulence relates to the presence of disturbance throughtout the flowing fluid throughout the entire oscillatory cycle, it is usually associated with the formation of eddies and vortices. However, the presence of vortices through part of the cycle, or in a specific location, does not mean that the flow is turbulent. This confusion appears in the majority of the medical publications about the subject. Other contributors to the formation of disturbances are the valves in the venous system, and the reversal of flow in segments of the arterial system. It is also possible that the oscillatory action of the precapillary sphincter contributes to disturbances in the flowing blood, that are sufficient to determine instability; this, however, was not established experimentally.

Experiments to observe this instability were carried out by many investigators, e.g., Helps and McDonald,[7] Hale et al.,[6] Yellin,[36] Nerem et al.,[19,20] Clark,[4] Sabbah and Stein,[23] and many others. In all of these works it was observed that the instability, defined by most of them as turbulence, is associated with a specific pathology such as valvular stenosis or local narrowing of the vessel. All of these cases will be discussed later, when the normal and pathological case of flow through heart valves and the formation of thrombus are to be considered.

REFERENCES

1. **Aperia, A.,** Haemodynamical studies, *Skand. Arch. Physiol.,* 83, 1, 1940.
2. **Atabek, M. B.,** Wave propagation through a viscous fluid contained in a tethered initially stressed orthtropic elastic tube, *Biophys. J.,* 8, 626, 1968.
3. **Bergel, D. M.,** The dynamic elastic properties of the arterial wall, *J. Physiol. (London),* 156, 458, 1961.
4. **Clark, C.,** Turbulent velocity measurements in a model of aortic stenosis, *J. Biomech.,* 9, 677, 1976.
5. **Dinnar, U.,** The role of the surrounding tissue in the propagation of waves through the arterial system, *TIT J. Life Sci.,* 5, 49, 1975.
6. **Hale, J. F., McDonald, D. A., and Womersley, J. R.,** Velocity profiles of oscillating arterial flow, with some calculation of viscous drag and the reynolds number, *J. Physiol.,* 128, 629, 1955.
7. **Helps, E. P. W. and McDonald, D. A.,** Observation on laminar flow in veins, *J. Physiol.,* 124, 631, 1954.
8. **Iberall, A. S.,** Attenuation of oscillatory pressures in instrument lines, U.S. Department of Commerce, Res. Paper RP2115, *J. Res. Nat. Bur. Stand.,* 45, 85, 1950.
9. **Iberall, A S.,** Study of the general dynamics of the physical chemical systems in mammals, *NASA Contract, Rep.,* 129, 1964.
10. **Lambert, J. W.,** On the nonlinearities of fluid flow in nonrigid tubes, *J. Franklin Inst.,* 266, 83, 1958.
11. **Lambossy, P.,** Oscillations force'es d'un liquide incompressible et viscueux dans un tube rigide et horizontal. Calcul de la force de frottement, *Helv. Phys. Acta,* 25, 311, 1952.
12. **Ling, S. C. and Atabek, H. B.,** A nonlinear analysis of pulsatile flow in arteries, *J. Fluid Mech.,* 55, 493, 1972.
13. **McDonald, D. A.,** *Blood Flow in Arteries,* Edward Arnold, London, 1974.
14. **McDonald, D. A. and Gessner, U.,** Wave attenuation in a visco-elastic arteries, in *Hemorheology,* Copley, A. L., Ed., Pergamon Press, Elmsford, N.Y., 1968, 113.
15. **Mersky, I.,** Wave propagation in a viscous fluid contained in an orthotropic elastic tube, *Biophys. J.,* 7, 165, 1967.
16. **Mones, A. I.,** *Die Pulskurue,* Leiden, 1878.

17. **Morgan, G. W. and Kiely, J. P.**, Wave propagation in a viscous liquid contained in a flexible tube, *J. Acoust. Soc. Am.*, 27, 715, 1954.

18. **Morgan, G. W. and Ferrante, W. R.**, Wave propagation in elastic tubes filled with streaming liquid, *J. Acoust. Soc. Am.*, 27, 715, 1955.

19. **Nerem, R. M., Steed, W. A., and Wood, N. B.**, An experimental study of the velocity distributions and transition to turbulence in the aorta, *J. Fluid Mech.*, 52, 137, 1972.

20. **Nerem, R. M., Pumberger, J., Gross, D., Hamlin, R. L., and Geiger, G. L.**, Hot-film anemometer velocity measurements of arterial blood flow in horses, *Circ. Res.*, 34, 193, 1974.

21. **Olsen, J. H. and Shapiro, A. H.**, Large-amplitude unsteady flow in liquid-filled elastic tubes, *J. Fluid Mech.*, 33, 513, 1967.

22. **Richardson, E. G. and Tyler, W.**, 1929, cited by Womersley, J. R., in Reference 34.

23. **Sabbah, H. N. and Stein, P. D.**, Effect of erythrocylic deformability upon turbulent blood flow, *Biorheology*, 13, 305, 1976.

24. **Schlicting, H.**, *Boundary Layer Theory*, McGraw-Hill, New York, 1960.

25. **Skalak, R. and Stathis, T.**, A porous tapered elastic tube model of a vascular bed, in *Biomechanics*, Fung, Y. C., et al., Eds., Prentice-Hall, Englewood Cliffs, N.J., 1966.

26. **Streeter, V. L., Keitzer, W. F., and Bohr, D. F.**, Pulsatile pressure and flow through distensible vessels, *Circ. Res.*, 13, 3, 1963.

27. **Streeter, V. L., Keitzer, W. F., and Bohr, D. F.**, Energy dissipation in pulsatile flow through distensible tapered tube, in *Pulsatile Blood Flow*, Attinger, E. V., Ed., McGraw-Hill, New York, 1964, 149.

28. **Taylor, M. G.**, An experimental determination of the propagation of fluid oscillations in a tube with visco-elastic wall, *Phys. Med. Biol.*, 4, 63, 1959.

29. **Uchida, S.**, The pulsating viscous flow superposed on the steady laminar motion of imcompressible fluid in a circular pipe, *Z. Angew. Math. Phys.*, 7, 403, 1956.

30. **Witzig, K.**, Uber Erzwungene Wellenbewegungen Zaher, Inkompressibler Flussigkeiten in Slastischen Rohren, Ph.D. Dissertation, University of Bern, Bern, 1914.

31. **Womersley, J. R.**, Oscillatory flow in arteries: effect of radial variation in viscosity on rate of flow, *J. Physiol.*, 127, 38, 1955.

32. **Womersley, J. R.**, Method for the calculation of velocity, rate of flow, and viscous drag in arteries when the pressure gradient is known, *J. Physiol.*, 127, 553, 1955.

33. **Womersley, J. R.**, Oscillatory motion of a viscous liquid in a thin-walled elastic tube. I. The linear approximation for long waves, *Philos. Mag.*, 46, 199, 1955.

34. **Womersley, J. R.**, The mathematical analysis of the arterial circulation in a state of oscillatory motion, Wright Air Development Center, Technical Report WADC-TR56—614, Dayton, 1957.

35. **Womersley, J. R.**, Oscillatory flow in arteries: the constrained elastic tube as a model of arterial flow and pulse transmission, *Phys. Med. Biol.*, 2, 178, 1957.

36. **Yellin, E. L.**, Laminar-turbulent transition process in pulsatile flow, *Circ. Res.*, 19, 791, 1966.

Chapter 7

ANALOG MODELS OF THE CIRCULATION

From the early days of scientific study of the human circulation system, investigators found it easier to refer to an analog model rather than the real system, and use the analog model to explain the behavior of the human system under varying conditions. The various models used by different investigators range from very simple to highly complex and sophisticated models. These models can be classified not only by their complexity, but also by the purpose they are designed to fulfill. This can range from easier explanations of the system for teaching purposes, such as the early circulatory model of Krogh,[9] to attempts at models that will yield mathematical relations to describe behavior and control of the system, which is the topic of this chapter.

The various mathematical models of the circulatory system can also be separated into different categories. The real analogs of the circulatory system are the models which replace the real body compartment, like vessel walls, blood, and even the various other blood constituents by either mechanical or electrical analogies, whose constitutive relations are well established. The other categories are the models which assume a system of mathematical expressions to represent the behavior of system components. The response of the real system is compared with the solution of this set of equations and used to improve the model. They, in turn, can be further divided according to the use assigned to the model.

The mathematical models can be used for one of the following classifications:

1. The formulation of mathematical relations that govern behavior of an isolated specific organ such as heart, kidney, etc.
2. The formulation of a mathematical expression of one specific parameter as function of the others, e.g., the cardiac output.
3. The incorporation of specific class of models into a gross model of the circulatory system or part of the system.
4. A formulation of theories that describe the interrelation between different system parameters. This class is usually aimed at obtaining an empirical relation.

Two additional types of mathematical models are found in the literature, however, they are different from the previous ones and are not to be considered here. These are the formulation of the interactions between the human body as a whole and the environment, and the development of mathematical procedure for the analysis of large quantities of data.

A legitimate question to be asked is, why is it at all necessary to use a mathematical or analog model, rather than deal with the actual system? The reason for this is the complexity of the real system; there are thousands of variables and factors that affect the properties, responses, and control of the human circulation. It is impossible to study all of them at the same time, or even to clearly define the contribution of specific variables to any specific observed phenomenon. It is even more complex as most of these variables interact with each other, and in some of them the knowledge of their specific task is not defined properly. In an analog model it is possible to abolish most of the parameters and to include only a few variables at a time. It is important to realize that because of this reason it is impossible to prove that the obtained relations are actually the complete description. Even if the results agree well with in vivo experiments the proof is not complete, since there is no evidence of the uniqueness of the solution. On the other hand an inclusion of all the parameters is equivalent to a study of the real system, and thus eliminates the efficiency of the analog model. Another advantage of using an analog model is in the prediction of extreme situations that are too dangerous to obtain in living systems.

The discussion in this chapter will concentrate on the basic techniques of modeling of the circulatory system, and as such will not review all the various models that appeared in the literature. The examples that are to be used are the ones which are widely accepted, and specific modeling of single organs or isolated segments are to be incorporated in the appropriate chapters.

A. The "Windkessel" Model

The earliest published mathematical analogy of the circulatory system appeared in 1899 by a German physiologist, Otto Frank. He suggested to represent the aorta and the proximal parts of the larger branches off the aorta by an elastic air-chamber with a uniform pressure and internal volume that is linearly proportional to this pressure. The name of this analog model is derived from the German words for air-chamber. Frank assumed that the rest of the circulation system can be replaced by a linear resistance. Further assumptions present in the model are negligible inertia and a pressure wavelength that is much larger than the characteristic length of the arterial system. Although this model is very simple and omits most of the system variables it can be found even in recent physiology textbooks as a representative model of the arterial system.

The basic assumption in the Windkessel model is the linear relation between pressure and volume. This assumption can be changed by a nonlinear one. However, the original Windkessel assumption was

$$V = CP \tag{1}$$

where V and P are the volume and pressure inside the air chamber, and C is the characteristic constant of proportionality. The fluid empties out of the air chamber into smaller size vessels where the flow is Poiseuille-type flow. It thus can be assumed that the rate of change of the internal volume is proportional to the driving pressure gradient. The pressure at the venous side of the system is assumed to be zero, thus enabling it to replace the driving pressure difference by the pressure inside the chamber. The constant of proportionality between volumetric rate of change, which equals the flow, and the pressure is the peripheral resistance, R.

$$\frac{dV}{dt} = \frac{P}{R} \tag{2}$$

This flow exists all the time. However, during systole there is an additional flow of fresh blood from the heart into the elastic chamber increasing both pressure and volume. The mathematical relations are given by:

$$\frac{dV}{dt} = Q_{in} = C\frac{dP}{dt} + \frac{P}{R} \tag{3}$$

where Q_{in} is the cardiac stroke and C is the capacitance of the system.

A schematic representation of the system is given in Figure 1. When the rate of flow into the aorta is known, Equation 3 can be solved to yield the pressure buildup in the chamber. The homogeneous solution of Equation 3 is given by

$$P_h = P_o \cdot e^{-t/Rc} \tag{4}$$

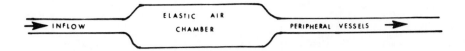

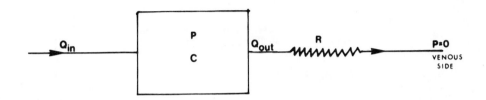

FIGURE 1. Conceptual model of the arterial circulation — the "Windkessel" model.

which upon insertion into Equation 3 yields in the following solution for the pressure

$$P = e^{-t/Rc}\left[P_0 + \frac{1}{c}\int_0^t e^{-\tau/Rc}\, Q_{in}\,(\tau)\,d\tau\right] \tag{5}$$

where P_o is to be determined by the condition of equal pulsation, namely

$$P\,(o) = P\,(T) = P_0 \tag{6}$$

As an example, when the cardiac output is taken as described in Figure 2, given by

$$Q_{in} = \begin{cases} Q_0 \sin\dfrac{2\pi t}{T} & 0 < t < T/2 \\[2mm] 0 & T/2 < t < T \end{cases} \tag{7}$$

the pressure pulse is obtained by direct integration to give:

$$P(t) = \left[P_0 + \frac{T}{2\pi}K\left(\frac{1}{Rc}\,Sin\,\frac{2\pi t}{T} - \frac{2\pi}{T}\,Cos\,\frac{2\pi t}{T}\right)e^{-t/Rc} + K\right]e^{-t/Rc} \tag{8a}$$

for $0 \leqslant t \leqslant T/2$, and

$$P(t) = \left[P_0 + K\left(1 + e^{T/2Rc}\right)\right]e^{-t/Rc} \tag{8b}$$

for $T/2 \leqslant t \leqslant T$, where P_o and K are constant given by:

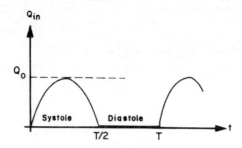

FIGURE 2.   An example of inflow (cardiac output) — half wave rectifier model.

$$K = \frac{2\pi}{CT} \cdot \frac{Q_o}{\left(\frac{1}{Rc}\right)^2 + \left(\frac{2\pi}{T}\right)^2}$$

$$\tag{9}$$

$$P_o = K \frac{e^{\frac{T}{2Rc}} + 1}{e^{\frac{T}{2Rc}} - 1}$$

It is thus clear that the results are linearly dependent on the rate of flow Q_o. The value of Q_o can be defined by integration of Q_{in} over the period and making the result equal the stroke volume. If the output of the heart is taken as 5 ℓ/min, the value of Q_o is given for the previous examples as $Q_o = 5000/60$ cm³/sec. An example for a specific set of parameters of the pressure wave is given in Figure 3. For this set of parameters the maximum value of pressure (systolic pressure) and the minimum value (diastolic pressure) are the criterion for the suitability of the parameters. In this example the pressures are 125/80 mmHg, the average found in the human population.

It is more convenient to describe Equation 3 by an electric analog, Figure 4. This electric circuit has the same differential equation, where current represents rate of flow and voltage represents pressure. This analog circuit permits the use of an analog computer to obtain various solutions for different sets of parameters. By the same way it can be represented by different mechanical analogs, according to the correspondences described in Table 1.

The electrical analog also enables, without any difficulty, the introduction of fluid inertia, by adding an inductance in series with the peripheral resistance as shown in Figure 5. However, it is clear in this example, that adding the inductance adds very little to the physiological knowledge, except that the additional term to the differential equation shows that this added term represents inertia.

The set of equations for this system is given by:

$$P = L\frac{dQ_1}{dt} + RQ_1$$

$$Q_2 = C\frac{dp}{dt} \tag{10}$$

$$Q_{in} = Q_1 + Q_2$$

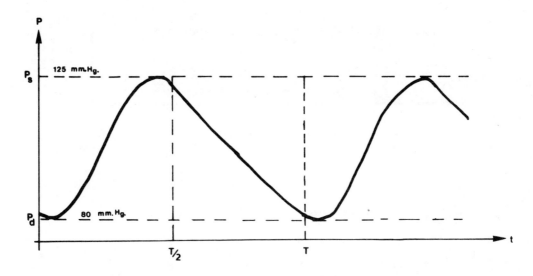

FIGURE 3.   The pressure pulse for the example described in the text. C-8.10⁻⁴ cm⁵/dyn; RC = 1.2 sec.; T = 1 sec. (60 b.p.m.)

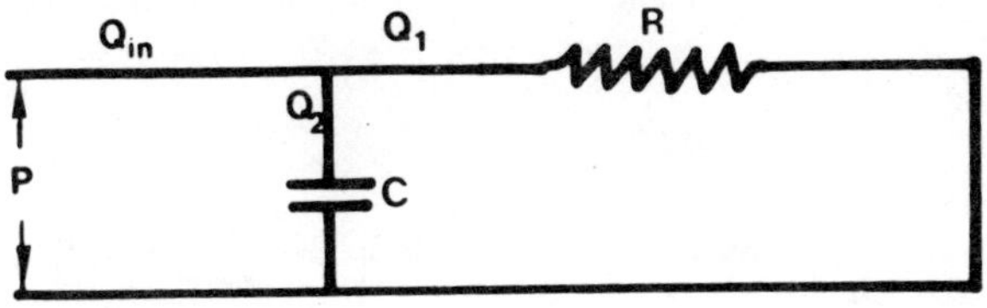

FIGURE 4.   Electrical analog of the "Windkessel" conceptual model.

Table 1
POSSIBILITIES FOR ANALOGS OF THE FLOW SYSTEM AND THEIR CORRESPONDENCES

Hydrodynamic system	Electrical analog	Mechanical analog	Mechanical analog
Pressure	Voltage	Force	Velocity
Volume flow	Current	Velocity	Force
Compliance	Capacitor	Spring	Mass
Fluid inertia	Inductance	Mass	Spring
Resistance to flow	Resistance	Dashpot	Dashpot

where the meaning of Q_1 and Q_2 is obvious from the figure, but no physiological meaning can be attributed to those parameters.

The set of equations can be reduced to a single second order differential equation

$$LC = \frac{d^2p}{dt^2} + RC \frac{dp}{dt} + P = L \frac{dQ_{in}}{dt} + RO_{in} \qquad (11)$$

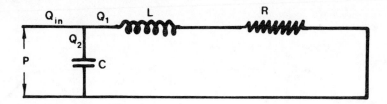

FIGURE 5.   Electrical analog of the "Windkessel" conceptual model with added element representing fluid inertia.

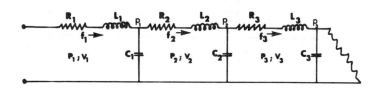

FIGURE 6.   Modified "Windkessel" model with added peripheral resistance, Rp.

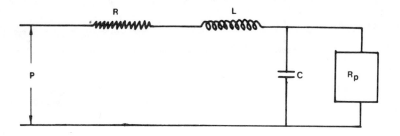

FIGURE 7.   Lumped-parameter model of an arterial segment, showing three compartments. The pressure inside each of the compartments is assumed uniform.

The type of solution for this equation depends on the relative values of $(RC)^2$ and 4 LC. However, in reality the value of fluid inertia is such that 4 LC is always larger than $(RC)^2$, which corresponds to a solution with small superimposed ripples. However, there is very little use for the gross model as shown in Figure 5. It is more useful to relate the analog to a single segment of the circulation, and combine this to a resistance representing the peripheral resistance, Figure 6.

Wesseling et al.[17] used this type of model for an arterial segment of the human arm. They related these parameters to blood properties (viscosity μ, and density ϱ) and wall geometry (length of vessel, ℓ, cross-sectional area S and radial/wall thickness ratio h), and vessel properties (Young's modulus E) by:

$$R = \frac{8 \pi \mu \ell}{S^2} \qquad \text{(Poiseuille flow)}$$

$$L = \frac{\rho \ell}{S} \qquad\qquad\qquad (12)$$

$$C = \frac{3 S (1 + h)^2}{E (1 + 2h)}$$

Typical values for such a segment are:

$$2r = 1 \text{ cm}; \quad \mu = 0.03 \text{ poise}; \quad \ell = 10 \text{ cm}; \quad = 1.06 \frac{\text{dyn} - \text{sec}^2}{\text{cm}^4}$$

$$h = 1/_{0.16} ; \quad E = 1.10^5 \text{ dyn}/_{\text{cm}^4}$$

which yield

$$C = 9.17 \cdot 10^{-4} \text{ cm}^5/\text{dyn} \tag{13}$$

$$L = 13.5 \frac{\text{dyn} - \text{sec}^2}{\text{cm}^5}$$

$$R = 12.22 \frac{\text{dyn} - \text{sec}}{\text{cm}^5}$$

which prove that indeed for each arterial segment 4 LC is much larger than $(RC)^2$, which leads to damping with vibration of the systolic pressure peak.

With the establishment of analog models of arterial segment, it is possible to reduce the size of the segment, and to add few segments together to represent a change in elastic properties, diameter, or other vessel properties. The result is a lumped parameter model, as shown in Figure 7. This leads to an increase of model accuracy, but the addition of more parameter adds to the uncertainty of the uniqueness of solutions. For the lumped parameters analog each compartment is specified by its pressure, P_i and volume, V_i and three analogous parameters: resistance to flow R_i, inductance L_i, and capacitance C_i. With these variables predefined for a specific arterial segment it is possible to calculate the current in each loop, which is analog to rate of flow f_i.

The equations for each of the segments can be written separately. Writing Ohm's law for junction i results in the following equations:

$$P_i - P_{i-1} = R_i f_i + L_i \frac{df_i}{dt}$$

$$P_i = \frac{V_i}{C_i} \tag{14}$$

$$f_i - f_{i-1} = \frac{dv_i}{dt}$$

Hence, the problem is reduced to a solution of a set of first-order differential equations. It is simpler to use an analog computer and to obtain results directly. It also allows for continuous change of parameters which enables an easier procedure for curve fitting. However, it is again not clear if a particular set of variables that fit a given result is the only set that yields this result, or there may be many more.

It is possible to expand this model further by allowing further branching at a specific junction. As an example consider the example of arteriovenous fistula used for kidney dialysis, shown in Figure 8. The hemodialysis process necessitates a vein of large caliber so that repeated puncture can be performed without accumulated damage. This is achieved by connecting the radial artery in the arm with an adjacent vein, thus creating a fistula with large quantities of blood flow in a large vessel. With S_{sh} open, Figure 8 represents the circulation analog of blood flow in the arm. The segment R_o, L_o, C_o represents the brachial artery, where $P_o(t)$ is the pressure wave approaching the arm from the aorta. The brachial artery bifurcates into the ulnar and radial arteries. The

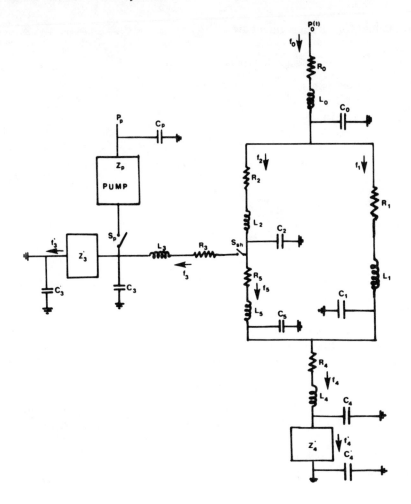

FIGURE 8.   Electrical analog of the arterial circulation in the arm of patient with arteriovenous fistula (when S_{sh} is closed) undergoing hemodialysis treatment (by closing switch Sp). Explanation of symbols is in the text.

radial artery is divided into two segments, according to the future insertion of the fistula. The two arteries combine into a set of two arches at the dorsal portion of the palm and then branches off to the various arteries inside the palm. This is represented by two segments. R_4, L_4, and C_4 represent the arches and the proximal parts of the branches. The peripheral arterioles and capillaries are combined to a peripheral segment with resistance Z_4' and capacitance C_4'. Ground represents the venous pressure, where it is assumed that pressure is very low and can be considered zero, without introduction of a too large error. Hence, the flow in the different segments prior to surgery can be calculated, or if known, serve to evaluate the various parameters.

With the formation of the shunt the switch S_{sh} is closed and additional segments that combine the shunted vein (R_3, L_3, and C_3) and the additional larger veins up to a point where pressure is actually zero (Z_3' and C_3') are added to the analog model. This situation represents the normal situation after surgery. When the patient undergoes hemodialysis treatment, a needle is inserted into the vein and a pump (usually roller pump) is added into the system, drawing given quantities of blood, passing them through the membranes and then returning them, usually at the same location, or into another vein. Thus the hemodialysis is introduced by closing the switch S_p.

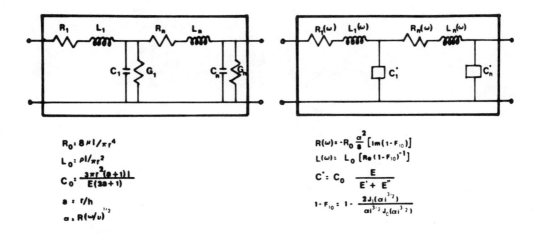

FIGURE 9. Four-terminal building blocks for arterial modeling. Left: frequency-independent parameters. Right: frequency-dependent parameters. In the expression for C* the symbols E′ and E″ stand for the real and imaginary parts of the complex elastic modulus while E* and E are the values of the frequency independent case. (From Attinger, E. O., *Advances in Biomedical Engineering and Medical Physics*, Vol. 1, Levine, S. N., Ed., Interscience, New York, 1968, 1. With permission.)

This example shows the relative ease of adopting an analog model for a given situation in any segment of the arterial tree. However, it is obvious from the figure that for this specific case 24 parameters, for which there is no knowledge about their values, must be predefined.

Further expansion of this model, or the previous model, can be achieved by introducing feedback control loop at control point. This feedback loop can be assigned control of either pressure or flow. This requires additional assumptions on the exact nature of the control and the interpretation of data. Examples of control loop are to be discussed later.

Beneken[3] used the basic scheme in Figure 7 to study the distribution of dye injected into the circulatory system. By assuming instantaneous and complete mixing of the substance it is possible to relate concentration and flow by using the continuity equation. This, however, relates to the blood flow measurement technique and is beyond the scope of the chapter.

Another modification of the basic element was suggested by many investigators, e.g., Noordergraaf et al.[12] and Wiener et al.[18] This basic element can be combined with the Womersley's solution discussed earlier, as described by Attinger[1] shown in Figure 9. The parameters are shown for a basic block, for both cases of frequency-independent and dependent cases. Noordergraaf et al.[11] used this model to model the entire circulatory system as shown in Figure 10. The theoretical analysis leading to this type of modified model is discussed in the next section.

B. Transmission Line Analogy

Consider an arterial segment, where the cross-sectional area is changing continuously downstream. It is assumed that the changes in cross sections are strictly geometric, and the contributions of distensibility of the vessel walls are relatively small. This condition is known as the tapering of the arteries, and is considered continuous so that it is possible to describe the changes in either cross section or diameter by a given equation. Thus for any control volume the net outflow must equal the rate of change of the control volume. This can be written as:

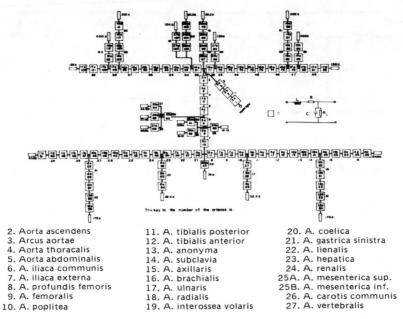

2. Aorta ascendens
3. Arcus aortae
4. Aorta thoracalis
5. Aorta abdominalis
6. A. iliaca communis
7. A. iliaca externa
8. A. profundis femoris
9. A. femoralis
10. A. poplitea

11. A. tibialis posterior
12. A. tibialis anterior
13. A. anonyma
14. A. subclavia
15. A. axillaris
16. A. brachialis
17. A. ulnaris
18. A. radialis
19. A. interossea volaris

20. A. coelica
21. A. gastrica sinistra
22. A. lienalis
23. A. hepatica
24. A. renalis
25A. A. mesenterica sup.
25B. A. mesenterica inf.
26. A. carotis communis
27. A. vertebralis

FIGURE 10.   Noordegraaf et al. model of the human circulatory system. Each box represents a segment of the arterial tree represented by the analog model shown in bottom. The top number in each box represents the segment notation (see key). The terminal boxes peripheral resistance. (From Noordegraaf, A., Verdouw, P. D., and Boom, H. B., *Prog. Cardiovasc. Dis.*, 5, 419, 1963. With permission.)

$$dQ = \frac{\partial Q}{\partial X} dX = -\frac{dV}{dt} = -\frac{\partial A}{\partial t} dX \tag{15}$$

where A is the cross-sectional area, X the longitudinal coordinate, Q the rate of flow, and V is the longitudinal velocity. This equation is true for any dX, thus, it yields

$$\frac{\partial A}{\partial t} + \frac{\partial Q}{\partial X} = 0 \tag{16}$$

The momentum equation with the inertial term and with negligible viscosity is given by

$$\frac{\partial U}{\partial t} + U \frac{\partial U}{\partial X} = \frac{1}{\rho} \frac{\partial P}{\partial X} \tag{17}$$

Since the viscosity effect is neglected, the velocity can be taken as uniform across the tube, so that it can be replaced by U = Q/A. With this relation Equation 16 can be divided by A, and Equation 17 by Q, so that when summed up together it gives

$$\frac{\partial Q}{\partial t} + \frac{\partial}{\partial X}\left(\frac{Q^2}{A}\right) = \frac{-A}{\rho} \frac{\partial P}{\partial X} \tag{18}$$

The second term is nonlinear, and is being eliminated in the analysis. Equation 18 is reduced to the following linear equation

$$\frac{\partial Q}{\partial t} + \frac{A}{\rho} \frac{\partial P}{\partial X} = 0 \tag{19}$$

The pressure is related to cross-sectional area by the distensibility of the blood vessel, which was referred to earlier as the capacitance of the system. The distensibility per unit length is defined as

$$C_u = \frac{\partial A}{\partial \rho} \tag{20}$$

The partial derivative is necessary since the cross section varies also with longitudinal distance. By this definition and Equation 16 the following relation is obtained

$$\frac{\partial Q}{\partial X} + C_u \frac{\partial P}{\partial t} = 0 \tag{21}$$

Equation 19 can be changed to a similar form, by the definition of inertance per unit length

$$L_u = \rho / A \tag{22}$$

So Equation 19 can be written as

$$\frac{\partial Q}{\partial t} + \frac{1}{L_u} \frac{\partial P}{\partial X} = 0 \tag{23}$$

Equations 21 and 23 are the basic set of equations for the flow in a tapering elastic tube with negligible inertia and viscosity. To describe more accurately the arterial system the small arterial branches can be considered as constant leakage throughout the entire length and through the arterial walls. This can be represented by a uniform leakage, characterized by a leakage resistance per unit length R_L. If the resistance of these branches is taken as R_B, these equations can be written for the more general as:

$$\frac{\partial Q}{\partial X} + C_u \frac{\partial P}{\partial t} = \frac{-P}{R_L}$$

$$\frac{\partial P}{\partial X} + L_u \frac{\partial Q}{\partial t} = -R_B Q \tag{24}$$

When the following analogy to an electrical circuit is used

Pressure = voltage	p	= V
Flow = current	Q	= i
Inertance = inductance	L_u	= L
Distensibility = capacitance	C_u	= C
Resistance to flow = resistance	R_B	= R

Equation 24 can be written in the following way:

$$\frac{\partial i}{\partial X} + C \frac{\partial V}{\partial t} = \frac{-V}{R_L}$$

$$\frac{\partial V}{\partial X} + L \frac{\partial i}{\partial t} = -Ri \tag{25}$$

These equations known in the literature as the Telegraph equations are the description of voltage and current in an electrical transmission line. Thus it is possible to use the well-established solution to these equations with the restriction that the structure of the cardivascular system is far more complex than the regular telegraph lines.

These two equations can be reduced to two second-order equations for each of the variables; written for the hydrodynamic case they are

$$\frac{\partial^2 P}{\partial X^2} - \left(\frac{1}{L_u} \frac{dL_u}{dX} \right) \frac{\partial P}{\partial X} - \frac{1}{C^2} \frac{\partial^2 P}{\partial t^2} = 0$$

(26)

$$\frac{\partial^2 Q}{\partial X^2} - \left(\frac{1}{C_u} \frac{dC_u}{dX} \right) \frac{\partial Q}{\partial X} - \frac{1}{C^2} \frac{\partial^2 Q}{\partial t^2} = 0$$

where C is given by the following relation

$$C = \left(\frac{1}{L_u C_u} \right)^{\frac{1}{2}}$$

(27)

and can be interpreted as the wave speed of propagation, or as defined by Taylor,[15] the nominal wave velocity.

Noordergraaf[11] used this equation in his analog model to include the four elements representing inductance, resistance, capacitance, and leakage resistance as shown at the bottom of Figure 10.

Looking at the nature of Equation 26 it is obvious that the equation will have constant coefficients only if both L_u and C_u are not a function of X. This will be the case in cylindrical tube. In the case of tapered tube the coefficients are a function of the longitudinal coordinate X.

Define a new variable Z_o, defined as the nominal characteristic impedance

$$Z_o = \left(\frac{L_u}{C_u} \right)^{\frac{1}{2}}$$

(28)

It is convenient to introduce a new parameter

$$\Omega = C \frac{d}{dX} (\ell n \, Z_o)$$

(29)

and a transformation of the longitudinal coordinate

$$S = \int_o^X \frac{dX}{C}$$

(30)

With these variables Equation 26 is transformed to the following equations:

$$\frac{\partial^2 P}{\partial S^2} - \Omega \frac{\partial P}{\partial S} - \frac{\partial^2 P}{\partial t^2} = 0$$

(31)

$$\frac{\partial^2 Q}{\partial S^2} + \Omega \frac{\partial Q}{\partial S} - \frac{\partial^2 Q}{\partial t^2} = 0$$

The variable Ω, called the taper parameter, determines the nature of the equations. For $\Omega = 0$ these equations are reduced to a simple wave equation, which is defined as a case of uniform transmission. In this special case Z_o the characteristic impedance is constant throughout the entire length. Another case where the solution is relatively simple is when Ω is independent on the variable S.

In this case the equations have uniform coefficients, and a solution can be obtained by simple Fourier analysis. Before solving the equations it is reasonable to establish the meaning of uniform taper factor. Consider a vessel with uniform elastic modulus and uniform ratio between vessel wall thickness and vessel diameter. An approximation for the characteristic impedance for this case is given by

$$Z_o{}^2 = \frac{\rho}{\pi R^2} \frac{E_h}{R^3} = C^\star \frac{1}{R^4} \tag{32}$$

or by

$$\ln Z_o = C_1 - 2 \ln R \tag{33}$$

where $C^\star$ and C_1 are constants. The nominal wave velocity for this case is also uniform, given by

$$C^2 = \frac{E_h}{2\pi\rho} \tag{34}$$

thus Equation 29 is reduced to

$$\Omega = C\left(-\frac{2}{R} \frac{dR}{dX}\right) = \text{constant} \tag{35}$$

which upon integration gives

$$R = R_o e^{-\frac{\Omega}{2C} X} \tag{36}$$

So the special case $\Omega = $ constant represents an elastic vessel of uniform elasticity and a radius which decreases exponentially from the vessels inlet, and with a constant ratio of vessel thickness to vessel diameter. For this case, as well as for the case of nonconstant parameters, the pressure and rate of flow can be assumed to be of the following form:

$$P = R_e \left(\sum_{n=0}^{\infty} P_n (S) e^{in\omega t}\right)$$

$$Q = R_e \left(\sum_{n=0}^{\infty} Q_n (S) e^{in\omega t}\right) \tag{37}$$

which upon introduction into Equation 31 gives the following solution (for constant Ω)

$$Q_n(S) = K_{1n} e^{\Upsilon_{1n}S} + K_{2n} e^{\Upsilon_{2n}S}$$

$$P_n(S) = K_{3n} e^{(\Upsilon_{1n} + \Omega)S} + K_{4n} e^{(\Upsilon_{2n} + \Omega)S}$$

(38)

where γ_{1n} and γ_{2n} are the roots of the equation

$$\Upsilon^2_{in} + \Omega \Upsilon_{in} + n^2 w^2 = 0$$

(39)

and K_{1n} and K_{4n} are constants. To determine these constants it is necessary to define the boundary conditions, and this is where the matching between the specific segment and the rest of the circulatory system comes into play. The matching conditions are rate of flow at the inlet $X = 0$ (which is the same as $S = 0$), and matched resistance, Z_o, at the outlet $X = 1$. The resistance at the outlet of the arterial system equals the peripheral resistance.

The difficulty in using this model is in choosing the right values for these impedances. However, there is an additional difficulty in most cases where there is a reflection at the terminal end. Only when both impedances are the same there is no reflection, in all other cases there is a reflection given by the relation obtained by Lewis and Wells[10] as

$$R_{(X=\ell)} = \frac{Z_T \left(1 + \frac{ic}{2\omega} \frac{\partial}{\partial X} \ell n\, Z_o \mid X=\ell \right) - Z_o}{Z_T \left(1 - \frac{ic}{2\omega} \frac{\partial}{\partial X} \ell n\, Z_o \mid X=\ell \right) + Z_o}$$

(40)

where Z_T is the terminal impedance. For large values of ω, the reflection coefficient approaches the value of the reflections obtained in a uniform line, and given by

$$R = \frac{Z_T - Z_o}{Z_T + Z_O}$$

(41)

Typical example for the modulus and phase of the impedance as a function of ω, based on this theory was calculated numerically by Taylor[15] and is described in Figure 11.

With the improvements in computer technology the need for this kind of model has diminished, and investigators were able to combine these models with control functions and demand and supply of various other quantities, like oxygen, or sugars, and others. This enables the modeling of larger systems and more variables, as is discussed in the following section.

C. Models of the Entire Circulatory System

The previous models are satisfactory when only a segment of the arterial tree is considered. Analysis of the entire system must include the whole body together with certain control capabilities. This requires introduction of control functions and additional elements like left ventricle, heart valves, valves in the venous system, stenotic areas, and many others. The mathematical description of these elements is too complex to be used in the previous mathematical models. It is also impossible to represent these functions by a simple electrical circuit, and new technique must be incorporated. It is convenient to use either mechanical or electrical analogs.

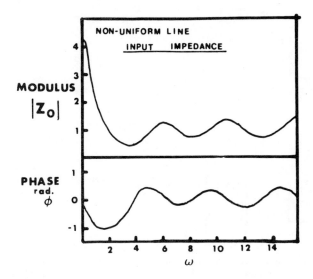

FIGURE 11. Modulus and phase of input impedance for nonuniform transmission line. For large values of W, both modulus and frequency fluctuate about the nominal value. (From Taylor, M. G., *Pulsatile Blood Flow*, McGraw-Hill, New York, 1964, 343. With permission.)

Although a mechanical analog is more clumsy, and much harder to satisfy all the nondimensional similarity characteristics, it is more appropriate for the study of artifical organs and valves. It is also suitable for the study of the nature of flow conditions. This model can provide information about the distribution of velocity across the tube, turbulence or vortex formation, points of separation of flow, etc. However, it is very difficult to choose the right elastic material in order to satisfy the similarity conditions defined by the flow conditions. It is because of this reason that most mechanical analogs are built with rigid walls, as for example the mechanical analog built by Osborn et al.[13] whose diagram and general view are shown in Figure 12, or the model developed by the group in Hydrospace Research Corp. in 1967 and known as the Mock Circulatory System. This analog model is currently used, with certain modifications, by many investigators for the study of artificial heart valves, artificial hearts, and different biomaterials. In all of these analog models the left ventricle is replaced by a flow pump (rather than by a pressure pump) and the pressures within the analog system are obtained by the values of the various peripheral resistances. The control of this pump and the peripheral resistances is extremely hard to achieve with a mechanical analog, and when these properties are to be analyzed it is easier to use an electrical analog.

In the electrical analog the left ventricle is represented by a generator with voltage pulse that is similar to the shape of the pressure input, and frequency controlled by a multivibrator. In the same way the valves can be represented by a diode in series with the inductor, or by a solenoid valves. Figure 13 shows an electrical analog of the same system designed by Osborn et al.[13] which is described by Figure 12.

With the advances in computer technology it is easier to describe these functions using a digital analog, as for example Fairchild et al.[6] In all of these models the cardiovascular control is composed of two separate components that are working with the same central control system. The autoregulation control employs the hemodynamic properties of the cardiovascular system and is directly related to peripheral resistance in different locations within the body. The other controls, which monitor chemical

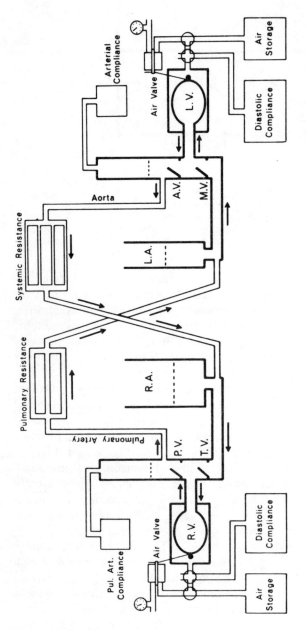

FIGURE 12.   Schematic diagram of mechanical circuit. (From Osborn, J. J., Hoehne, W., and Badia, W., *Physical Bases of Circulatory Transport, Regulation and Exchange*, W. B. Saunders, Philadelphia, 1967, 47. With permission.)

and hormonal changes within the body, control the heart load and therefore the heart rate. It is, however, normal that a deviation from set valves in one control system will trigger the other system.

The input to all the models is by the work load demand. This consists of two components: one is the load of maintenance of the body, while the other is defined by the type of activity. Both these demands are translated by the body to required oxygen supply. Extra activity in any part of the body affects peripheral resistance in two ways. The local control which monitors a temporary lack of oxygen will locally constrict the blood vessel causing an increase in peripheral resistance, at the same time (or even before there is a local lack of oxygen) the central nervous system, by anticipation of work load demand, will constrict the vessel via the vasomotor nerves. This change in peripheral resistance causes an increase in blood pressure which is continuously monitored by the carotid sinus baroreceptors. Upon deviation of arterial blood pressure from a set pressure reference a signal is transferred to the central nervous system, which in turn by a nervous command produces a change in heart action that includes both heart rate and cardiac output. Hence, the action of the heart is regulated in such a way that keeps the arterial blood pressure stable, and minimizes the amount of fluctuations.

In cases where the excessive load is too high, there will be a rise in arterial pressure despite this regulatory control. However, this pressure will decline back to normal with the disappearance of the excess work load demand. An analog representation of these mechanisms can be built by a detailed model that determines the force of contraction, the propagation of contraction wave (conduction system of the cardiac muscle) and many other parameters. Such a model was suggested by De Pater and Den Berg[5] which includes generators representing heart muscle action with tension developed by the duration, shape, and amplitude of the contraction wave, Figure 14, which sends signals to a system of capacitors with values equal to cardiac chamber volume and vessel resistances similar to those discussed earlier, Figure 15. It is, however, possible to use a simple model that does not include the cardiac mechanical details and relates only cardiac output, Q, to heart rate F, and stroke volume S_v, by the simple relation

$$Q = F.S_v \qquad (42)$$

Since the heart operates as a flow pump, rather than a pressure pump, the cardiac output determines the developed pressure difference between the arterial and venous sides. The venous pressure is very small compared with the mean arterial pressure and can be omitted with only very small error. Thus the arterial pressure is defined by the total peripheral resistance by the linear relations:

$$P = Q.R_p \qquad (43)$$

where R_p is the total peripheral resistance, which includes both small and large arteries together with the microcirculation in the capillaries.

This pressure, as was discussed earlier, is compared with the set reference pressure and serves as a feedback control to both heart rate and total peripheral resistance. There is a lack of knowledge as to exact transfer function for this feedback. Warner[16] assumed that the transfer function is a linear function of the actual pressure difference and the rate of arterial pressure changes.

$$e_1 = K_1 (P - P_s) + K_2 \frac{dP}{dt} \qquad (44)$$

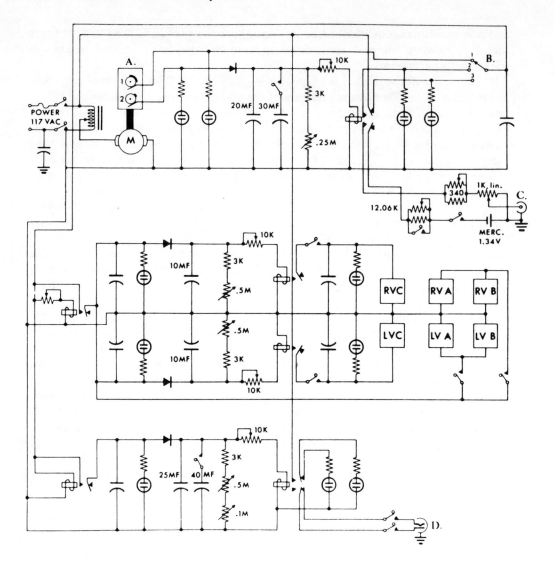

FIGURE 13.   Schematic diagram of electrical circuit. (From Osborn, J. J., Hoehne, W., and Badia, W., *Physical Bases of Circulatory Transport, Regulation and Exchange,* W. B. Saunders, Philadelphia, 1967, 47. With permission.)

where e_1 is the carotid sinus nerve signal rate of discharge. P_s is the set reference point and K_1, K_2 are constants. This same idea was expanded by Beneken[2] for each of six chambers representing pulmonary and systemic arterial and venous segments. This signal releases a stimulus that affects the cardiac rate, if the rate of discharge at the central nervous system is linear with respect to this signal, the heart rate function will be given by an integral of the carotid sinus nerve signal, or

$$e_2 = K_3 \int_0^t e_1 \, dt \tag{45}$$

where e_2 is the error-correcting function of heart rate, or the transfer function between

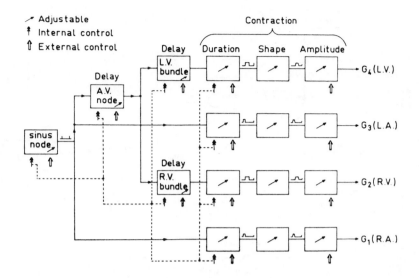

FIGURE 14. Analog model of the innervation of the heart. (From De Pater, L. and Den Berg, V., *Med. Electron. Biol. Eng.,* 2, 161, 1964. With permission.)

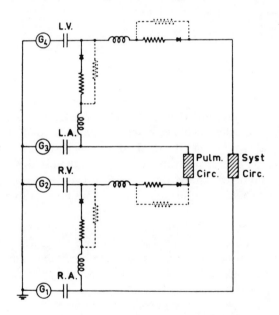

FIGURE 15. Analog model of the ventricles, the atria and the valves. (From De Pater, L. and Den Berg, V., *Med. Electron. Biol. Eng.,* 2, 161, 1964. With permission.)

the arterial pressure baroreceptors and the cardiac rate. In the same time the central nervous control responds to the change in pressure by a vasomotor activity that either constricts or dilates the peripheral vessels to change the peripheral resistance. These changes are superimposed on the changes that occurred earlier due to anticipation of blood flow demands that are determined by the type of activity. Because of this it is not a straightforward result of the carotid sinus nerve signal, e_1, but rather a complex unknown function of e_1 and the type of activity. What further complicates the analysis

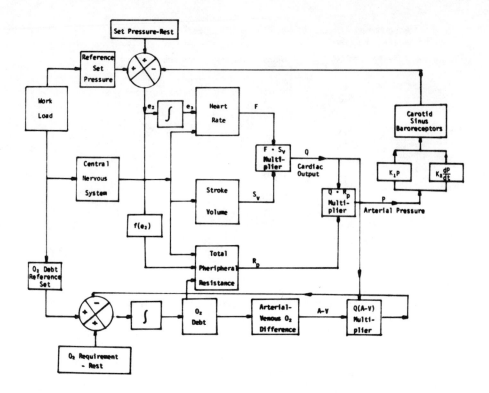

FIGURE 16.   Control diagram of cardiac output.

is the difference in time between these two signals, one with almost no time lag and the other with relatively long time delay. Pickering et al.[14] assumed for this control element a transfer function that includes a direct response to load together with a pure time delay that responds to the load demand; all of this is further subjected to a first-order time lag. This type of transfer function requires the use of four parameters, of which there is no physiological knowledge. It is, however, an assumption that can be used to obtain a given behavior of the entire system, but no guarantees for the uniqueness of the solution.

Another unknown is the anticipation control. Here again a set of parameters can be obtained to give the desired response, but again with no guarantees for uniqueness of the solution. It is because of this reason that the block diagram, shown in Figure 16 does not provide a specific transfer function, and only gives an arbitrary transfer function.

The system described so far is for the mechanical control part that controls arterial pressure. This system is controlled simultaneously by the chemical control elements that monitor oxygen deficiencies and arterial-venous oxygen differences. Here again the exact mechanism and especially the mathematical description of the control functions is not well established, there is, however, general agreement that the control is achieved by a neural error signal. The controlled variable in this case is the peripheral resistance, that is under vasomotor control. The error signal is obtained in response to oxygen debt by local and overall chemoreceptors activity. Again in this case, as was the case with pressure, the reference set point which is the oxygen requirement for rest is changed by anticipation of work load demand. This reference set value is compared with the oxygen debt obtained according to Fick's law by multiplying the arterial-venous oxygen difference and the cardiac output. However, this is not the only change in the cardiovascular system obtained due to oxygen debt. Another response to oxygen deficiency is increased breathing that changes the intrathoracic pressure condition, and, therefore, the venous return and the venous pressure. As a response to all this the heart rate is also changed, in an unknown function. The general model described so far is the basic control model, as shown in Figure 16. Various models based on this basic model appeared in the literature. The difference between these models is the different functions assumed for the relation between the parameters. As there is no general agreement as to the exact form of these transfer functions it is not discussed further. An example for models of this nature can be found in Pickering et al.,[14] and in the proceedings of an ISA meeting,[8] especially the model suggested by Croston et al.[4]

As was mentioned earlier the easiest way to handle this unknown transfer function is by using a digital computer analog. Since the possibilities for different functions, and as a result the number of different such models that appeared in the literature, are enormous, there is no reason to summarize them in this text.

REFERENCES

1. Attinger, E. O., Analysis of pulsatile blood flow, in *Advances in Biomedical Engineering and Medical Physics,* Vol. 1, Levine, S. N., Ed., Interscience, New York, 1968, 1.
2. Beneken, J. E. W., A Mathematical Approach to Cardio-Vascular Function: The Uncontrolled Human System, Ph.D. thesis, University of Utrecht, The Netherlands, 1965.
3. Beneken, J. E. W., Some computer models in cardiovascular research, in *Cardiovascular Fluid Dynamics,* Bergel, D. H., Ed., Academic Press, New York, 1972, 173.
4. Croston, R. C., Rummel, J. A., and Kay, F. J., Computer model of cardiovascular control system response to exercise, in *Regulations and Control in Physiological System,* Iberall, A. S. and Guyton, A. C., Eds., Instrument Society of America, Pittsburgh, 1973, 363.
5. De Pater, L. and Den Berg, V., An electrical analgoue of the entire human circulatory system, *Med. Electron. Biol. Eng.,* 2, 161, 1964.
6. Fairchild, B. T., Korvetz, L. J., and Huckaba, C. E., Digital computer simulation of arterial blood flow, in *Chemical Engineering in Medicine and Biology,* Hershey, D., Ed., Plenum Press, New York, 1967, 3.
7. Frank, O., Die Grundform des Arteriellen Pulses. Erste Abhandlung. Mathematische Analyse, *Z. Biol.,* 37, 483, 1899.
8. Iberall, A. S. and Guyton, A. C., Eds., *Regulation and Control in Physiological Systems,* Instrument Society of America, Pittsburgh, 1973.
9. Krogh, A., The regulation of the supply of blood to the right heart (with a description of a new circulation model), *Skand. Arch. Physiol.,* 27, 227, 1912.
10. Lewis, I. A. D. and Wells, F. H., *Millimicrosecond Pulse Techniques,* 2nd ed., Pergamon Press, Oxford, 1959.
11. Noordergraaf, A., Verdouw, P. D., and Boom, H. B., The use of analog computer in a circulation model, *Prog. Cardiovasc. Dis.,* 5, 419, 1963.
12. Noordergraaf, A., Verdouw, P. D., van Brummelen, A. G. W., and Wiegel, F. W., Analog of the arterial bed, in *Pulsatile Blood Flow,* Attinger, E., Ed., McGraw-Hill, New York, 1964, 373.
13. Osborn, J. J., Hoehne, W., and Badia, W., Ventricular function in the basic regulation of the circulation: studies with a mechanical analog, in *Physical Bases of Circulatory Transport, Regulation and Exchange,* Reeve, E. B. and Guyton, A., Eds., W. B. Saunders, Philadelphia, 1967, 47.
14. Pickering, W. D., Nikiforuk, P. N., and Merriman, J. E., Analogue computer model of the human cardiovascular control system, *Med. Biol. Eng.,* 7, 401, 1969.
15. Taylor, M. G., Wave travel in arteries and the design of the cardiovascular system, in *Pulsatile Blood Flow,* Attinger, E., Ed., McGraw-Hill, New York, 1964, 343.
16. Warner, H. R., The use of an analog computer for analysis of control mechanisms in the circulation, *Proc. IRE,* 47, 1913, 1959.
17. Wesseling, K. H., DeWaal, B. M. J., De Wit, B., and Beneken, J. E. W., Arm arterial parameters from externally measured pulsewave contours, as cited in Beneken.[3]
18. Wiener, F., Morkin, E., Skalak, R., and Fishman, A. P., Wave propagation in the pulmonary circulation, *Circ. Res.,* 19, 834, 1966.

Chapter 8

THE HEART AS A PUMP

A. Introduction

The heart, composed of two atria and two ventricles, is a combination of two synchronized pulsatile pumps in series. The synchronization of these four chambers is achieved by the cardiac muscle, which is a single triggering mechanism. The anatomy of the heart and a description of the cardiac events were discussed in Chapter 2. In this chapter, the heart, and especially the left ventricle, is discussed by considering its pumping activity. It is necessary to define, *a priori*, the exact mechanism of the cardiac pump, and to answer the question about the nature of its action: is the cardiac pump a constant pressure or a constant volume system? In other words, does the left ventricle push blood to the aorta up to a present systolic pressure, or is the amount of the cardiac stroke predefined and the aortic pressure is the dependent variable?

The inlet into the cardiac pump, the right atria, receives blood continuously from the great veins. This blood flows into the ventricle by two mechanisms: direct flow (approximately 70%) and by atrial contraction (additional 30%). Thus the amount of blood that enters the left ventricle is determined by the venous return, atrial contraction, and Starling mechanism. This volume, when inside the left ventricle, determines the volume of the ventricle and thus the length of the muscle fibers at the beginning of contraction. When contraction, due to excitation of muscle cells, takes place, the aortic valve is closed. Hence, the contraction is independent of arterial pressure, and the final ventricular volume at the end of contraction depends only on the initial ventricular volume and the characteristics of muscle contraction. Since blood is incompressible, the difference between these two volumes must be transmitted into the circulatory tree, through the aorta, thus increasing the pressure in the aorta. The subsequent systolic pressure is determined by this cardiac stroke and the mechanical characteristics of the systemic circulation (resistance, rheological properties of blood, and blood vessels) as was discussed in the previous chapters. Hence, it can be concluded that the heart is a constant volume pump. Because of this reason the performance of the heart as a pump can be described by the end diastolic volume, ventricular filling, and the contractile activity of the heart as a muscle. These parameters, which depend on many other parameters, can solely characterize the efficiency of the pumping activity.

It sounds simple, however, the measurement of these parameters, especially the contractile activity, is very complex, and interpretation of the results into quantitative descriptors is even more complex. To add to this, there is a disagreement and wide differences in the definitions of the various parameters used by many investigators to describe levels of activity and efficiency of the heart. A survey of the literature will reveal different descriptions of the dynamic activity of the heart and determination of pumping efficiency. This is more significant when these descriptions are incorporated into empirical formulation that sometimes are untrue and meaningless.

It is of utmost importance to be specific about the meaning of the terminology used, the exact interpretation of measurements and the precise definition of the mathematical modeling of the various elements.

B. Definition of Cardiac Parameters

The performance of the heart can be measured and characterized by the use of various mechanisms that contribute to its function. These parameters can be chemical, electrical, mechanical, or hydrodynamical, however, all of them are related to each other by the characteristics of the cardiac muscle, systemic circulation, and control mechanism. The interrelation of these mechanisms are either not fully understood or too complex to be of practical clinical application.

For many years different investigators used each one of these methods to arrive at some empirical criterions for cardiac performance, and especially at empirical values to define states in a failing heart. As a good illustration of such empirical relations, that appear as an empirical catalog, can serve any textbook of clinical cardiology, where measurement of action potential generation and ventricular conduction are recorded is the electrocardiogram (ECG), used to define deviation from the electrical behavior of normal sinus rhythm. The deviations from the normal pattern are used to define cardiac muscle and/or neuromuscular pathology.

The use of specific methods and parameters goes hand-in-hand with the advancement of technology and the introduction of newer measurement techniques. In an attempt to find suitable parameters for left ventricular performance, cardiologists have moved from values that relate only to blood pressure in the systemic circulation to values that combine blood pressure in the ventricle and in the systemic circulation with volumes of blood pumped by the heart. Lately the use of new parameters has given much better criteria for pumping efficiency, with the introduction of volume measurements by cineradiography, videometry, ultrasonic techniques, and real time stress-strain measurement in the ventricular wall by indirect techniques. The various indexes used can be described chronologically, however, it is more efficient to describe them according to the nature of the measurement used to arrive at this parameter.

1. Ventricular Volumes

The interpretation of the rate of change of ventricular volume is still complex, even with the advanced technology of three-dimensional visualization. It is because of this reason that even today, the suitable parameters are only static ventricular volume at specific cardiac events. They include:

End-Diastolic-Volume (EDV, Ved) — The volume of blood in the ventricle at the end of diastole. The normal value of EDV at rest is 120 to 150 mℓ. However when, due to a variety of conditions, the flow of blood during diastole into the ventricle increases, this value can get as high as 200 mℓ or more.

End-Systolic Volume (ESV, Ves) — The volume of blood in the ventricle at the end of systole. This parameter depends very strongly on the strength of cardiac muscle contraction. Its normal value at rest is 50 to 70 mℓ, but with very strong contraction more blood flows into the aorta, and the remaining blood volume at the end of systole can be as low as 10 to 30 mℓ.

Stroke-Volume (Vs) — The difference between end diastolic and end systolic volumes or the amount of blood pumped by the left ventricle into the aorta per beat. This parameter can be, in extreme situations, as low as a few milliliters, and can reach in trained athletes with a large heart values of 200 mℓ or more. The normal resting value is 70 to 80 mℓ.

The value of EDV, defined earlier, depends on the amount of blood that flows through the venous system. Usually, the potential volume of the left ventricle is not fully filled with blood, as there is a reserve volume to accommodate an increase in venous return. Thus another volume is sometimes used to define cardiac pumping efficiency. Diastolic-Reserve-Volume (DRV) the space of the ventricle at the end of diastole not occupied with blood.

Although the definitions are written for the left ventricle and might have instantaneous different values in the right ventricle, they are on the average equal due to Starling's law of the heart, as discussed in Chapter 2.

2. Pressure Parameters

Not like the volume parameters, the pressure measurement is continuous, so that the parameters can be either discrete or continuous. The pressure characteristics are used in two different ways. The first method uses the aortic pressures, which are easy to measure, and combines them with other variables to arrive at derived indices that determine cardiac load and other such general indices. This will be discussed later. The second approach is to combine left ventricular pressure and gradients with an analytical model for the ventricle during contraction to arrive at parameters that will give a criterion for left ventricular wall stress and contraction efficiency.

Aortic Pressure — Pressure measured at the roof of the aorta. In most cases this pressure is not measured directly at the root of the aorta, but in other places along the peripheral arteries. Usually, this pressure is measured by auscultatory method in the brachial artery and is considered to equal the pressure at the root of the aorta. This is not completely true as the effect of kinetic energy, which amounts to 2 to 3 mmHg, is not present at the brachial artery, as well as the effect of pressure wave attenuation that might reach few mmHg. The aortic pressure is represented by its highest and lowest values, the systolic and diastolic pressures, respectively, and the average aortic pressure defined as

$$\text{Pav} = \overline{P} = \frac{1}{3} \left(P \text{ diastole } + 2 P \text{ systole}\right) \tag{1}$$

Ventricular Pressure — The pressure inside the left ventricle. This pressure is recorded with a catheter inserted into the left ventricle, thus assuming that the pressure is equal throughout the ventricle, an assumption that neglects the kinetic energy of contraction. From this continuous measurement the first and second derivatives of the pressure can be obtained, either by direct differentiating or by numerical analysis of the recording. From this the following parameters are obtained:

1. Ventricular End Diastolic Pressure (VEDP) — The pressure in the left ventricle at the end of diastole.
2. Maximum Left Ventricular dp/dt — The peak rate of change of ventricular pressure.
3. Maximum Left Ventricular d^2p/dt^2 — The maximum second derivative of the ventricular pressure which is a good descriptor for the shortening of cardiac muscle fibers.

The last two parameters are used to describe the mechanical behavior of the cardiac muscle and are combined with analytical models to yield criterions for muscle contractile efficiency, as will be discussed later.

3. Hydrodynamic Parameters

The hydrodynamic parameters include both flow conditions, (e.g., turbulence, secondary flow, etc.) in both ventricles and the aorta, and flow characteristics, mainly velocity. Both of these descriptions are essential to describe the flow field which is of utmost importance in the diagnosis of pathological heart values or in the evaluation of blood supply to the cardiac muscle via the coronary arteries. They are less important in the evaluation of cardiac efficiency, since the nature of flow requires that only average values can be used. However, they are used in the analytical evaluation of contractility and as parameters in the derivation of cardiac load. The major hydrodynamic parameter is:

Ejection Velocity — The velocity of the blood pumped by the left ventricle as it enters the aorta. This velocity is a function of geometry and therefore refers only to the average velocity, thus sometimes defined as the mean systolic ejection velocity. The derivative of this velocity gives the acceleration of the blood and is used in the determination of cardiac pumping efficiency; since this quantity changes with time it is customary to take the peak rate of change of flow, or the maximum of flow derivative.

4. Mechanical Parameters

The mechanical descriptions used in various textbooks and other published works hide in themselves the assumption on the nature of cardiac muscle performance. This assumption, in some cases, is used without intention, and sometimes even in the wrong context. When the mechanical descriptors used are force, velocity, and length, the underlying assumption is a unidimensional performance of the cardiac muscle. This is used mainly to describe experimental finding, but they must include specifications of the direction of measurement, reference for velocity measurement and initial length, or changes in length between predefined points. If the assumption is that the cardiac muscle behaves as an elastic container the consideration should be that of three dimensional; and force, velocity, and length are not appropriate. Instead the consideration of stress, strain, and strain rate is required. A measurement of these quantities is not only complex and highly dangerous, but it requires simultaneous measurement at numerous places on the left ventricle. In addition the transformation of these measurements into a workable set of parameters that can serve as indices for cardiac efficiency or as descriptors of contractility is very hard. It is because of these reasons that the mechanical descriptors used most commonly to describe these parameters are based on specific models of cardiac muscle performance. Although the descriptors obtained in this way are known to be average quantities that are not directly measurable, they are very useful since they can be combined analytically to the other parameters described earlier. The descriptor used more often than others is:

Contractile Element Shortening Velocity, (Vce) — The definition of this term is neither straightforward nor simple, as it has no anatomical reality that can be measured. Instead it is based on a mathematical analog for the mechanism of cardiac muscle contraction. This analog assumes a one-dimensional response of the muscle to a force in the same direction. When the muscle is activated it generates force as it contracts. This force depends on the excitation of muscle cells which relates to velocity of shortening of the initial muscle length. The force generated by the muscle can be controlled by attaching a different afterload to the initial preload of the muscle specimen. The afterload should be added without a change in muscle length. Electrical stimulation is then applied to muscle, till the force generated is sufficient to raise the load. The velocity of shortening is recorded at this instant. This is done for different preloads and different initial lengths and the results are recorded and interpolated to zero load (preload and afterload), Figure 1. The extrapolated velocity for zero load converges for all the specimen to the same value, the maximal velocity of shortening (V_{max}), a result that was first discovered by Sonnenblick.[13] The determination of V_{max} is obtained by the use of Hill's equation, which relate the force P to the velocity v.

$$\text{Hill}^9 \quad (P + a)\, v_{ce} = b\,(Po - P) \qquad (2)$$

where a and b are functions of muscle fiber length, with the first representing rate of heat production during the contraction, the later the rate (absolute value) of energy liberation; and Po is the maximum force that the muscle is capable of producing. Fung[6] modified this equation to account for the time delay to reach the maximum force, by adding a power relation

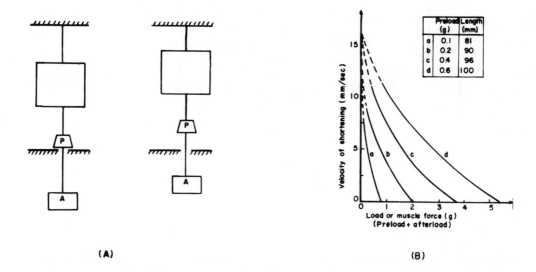

(A)

(B)

FIGURE 1. Afterloaded isotonic experiment. (A) Schematic outline. P represents the preload, and afterload A is added and the muscle is stimulated to shorten and carry the preload and afterload. (B) The force velocity relation for this experiment for different preloads and initial length. (From Pollack, G. H., *Circ. Res.*,26, 111, 1970. With permission.)

$$(P + a) v_{ce} = b (Po - P)^n ; \quad 0 < n < 1 \tag{3}$$

However, from Figure 1 it can be seen that the force-velocity relations are different for different initial length and preload. To consider this change various mechanisms of cardiac contraction have been proposed. All of these models contain a series elastic element (SE), a parallel elastic element (PE), together with a contractile element (CE). The arrangement of these three elements can be different as shown in Figure 2. However, in all of these models the expression of the velocity of shortening of the contractile elements depends on the force-velocity and length-velocity relations of the elastic and parallel elements. These quantities can be measured in an isolated heart, by various arrangements but are unknown in the intact heart. As an example for the expression for the shortening velocity, the most common models of Maxwell and Voigt models are considered by the method described by Hefner and Brown[8] and Pollack.[12]

a. Maxwell Model

In the arrangement of Maxwell body, Figure 2, the force acting on the series elastic (SE) and the contractile element (CE) is the same, and the sum of the deformation in both of them must be the same as that of the parallel element (PE). To make the results more general the force can be divided by the cross section of the muscle, and thus having a relation between stresses rather than forces. This is not completely true, but is used in all the textbooks and publications. With these assumptions the following relations can be written:

$$\sigma = \sigma_{SE} + \sigma_{PE} \tag{4}$$

$$\epsilon = \epsilon_{PE} = \epsilon_{SE} + \epsilon_{CE} \tag{5}$$

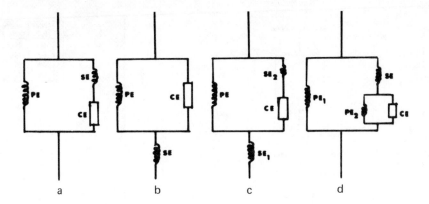

FIGURE 2.   Mechanical analog models for cardiac muscle.

where σ is the stress and ε is the strain of the corresponding elements. To obtain velocities, Equation 5 can be differentiated with respect to time, to yield:

$$\frac{d\epsilon}{dt} = \frac{d\epsilon_{SE}}{dt} + \frac{d\epsilon_{CE}}{dt} = \frac{d\epsilon_{SE}}{dt} - v_{CE} \tag{6}$$

The term $d\epsilon_{CE}/dt$ is not measurable during the experiment, but with the following relation:

$$\frac{d\epsilon_{SE}}{dt} = \frac{d\epsilon_{SE}}{d\sigma_{SE}} \cdot \frac{d\sigma_{SE}}{dt} = \left(\frac{d\sigma_{SE}}{d\epsilon_{SE}}\right)^{-1} \cdot \frac{d\sigma_{SE}}{dt} \tag{7}$$

it is possible to express this term by the stiffness of the series element (the last term in the equation), and the expression $d\sigma_{SE}/dt$ which can be written as

$$\frac{d\sigma_{SE}}{dt} = \frac{d\sigma}{dt} - \frac{d\sigma_{PE}}{dt} = \frac{d\sigma}{dt} - \frac{d\sigma_{PE}}{d\epsilon} \cdot \frac{d\epsilon}{dt} \tag{8}$$

where the expression $d\sigma_{PE}/d\varepsilon$ can be obtained by subjecting the specimen to various preloads, for which the contractile element and the series elasticity are neutral. Thus the velocity of shortening of the contractile element for Maxwell body is given by the following

$$v_{CE} = \frac{d\sigma/dt}{d\sigma_{SE}/d\epsilon_{SE}} - \frac{d\epsilon}{dt}\left(1 + \frac{d\sigma_{PE}/d\epsilon}{d\sigma_{SE}/d\epsilon_{SE}}\right) \tag{9}$$

where all the terms are measurable, part of them during the test and the other part before the test in the unstimulated muscle.

In the last equation there are two distinguished cases, the isometric contraction in which there is no change in length, corresponds to $d\varepsilon/dt = 0$ for which the equation reduces to

$$v_{CE} = \frac{d\sigma/dt}{d\sigma_{SE}/d\epsilon_{SE}} \tag{10}$$

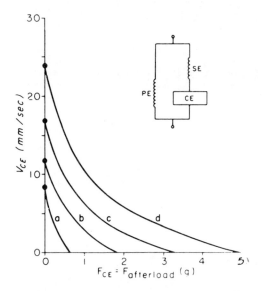

FIGURE 3. Force-velocity relations for a Maxwell body model. (From Pollack, G. H., *Circ. Res.*, 26, 111, 1970. With permission.)

and the case of isotonic contraction or isotonic shortening where the muscle generates a constant force, corresponds to $d\sigma/dt = 0$. For the later cases the equation reduces to

$$v_{CE} = \frac{-d\epsilon}{dt} \left(1 + \frac{d\sigma_{PE}/d\epsilon}{d\sigma_{SE}/d\epsilon_{SE}} \right) \tag{11}$$

which relates the velocity of shortening of the contractile element and the velocity of the muscle itself.

An example of the results obtained by Pollack[12] is given in Figure 3. The analytical expression for the isometric contraction shows that for a specific muscle the velocity of shortening is directly proportional to the rate of change of stress, and there is no correction for the transfer of load to the parallel element. In the isotonic contraction the velocity of shortening is higher than the muscle velocity by a coefficient that depends on the ratio of the stiffness of the parallel and elastic elements.

b. Voigt Model

The Voigt model has the same components as the Maxwell model, but in a different arrangement, Figure 2. In this model the force on the SE element, equals the sum of the forces acting of the PE and CE elements. The total elongation is also different from that obtained for the Maxwell model.

$$\sigma = \sigma_{SE} = \sigma_{PE} + \sigma_{CE} \tag{12}$$

$$\epsilon = \epsilon_{SE} + \epsilon_{CE} = \epsilon_{SE} + \epsilon_{PE} \tag{13}$$

Differentiating Equation 13, and using the same procedure described for the Maxwell model, yields the following expression:

$$\frac{d\epsilon}{dt} = \frac{d\epsilon_{SE}}{dt} - v_{CE} = \frac{d\epsilon_{SE}}{d\sigma} \cdot \frac{d\sigma}{dt} - v_{CE} \tag{14}$$

from this expression the velocity of shortening is obtained as

$$v_{CE} = \frac{d\sigma/dt}{\frac{d\sigma}{d\epsilon_{SE}}} - \frac{d\epsilon}{dt} \tag{15}$$

and for the two special cases of isometric contraction ($d\epsilon/dt = 0$) and isotonic contraction ($d\sigma/dt = 0$), the velocity of shortening is given by:

$$v_{CE} = \frac{d\sigma/dt}{d\sigma/d\epsilon_{SE}} \quad \text{isometric contraction}$$

$$\tag{16}$$

$$v_{CE} = -\frac{d\epsilon}{dt} = v_{muscle} \quad \text{isotonic contraction}$$

In this case the velocity of shortening, for the isotonic contraction, is the same as the muscle velocity, and as such can be measured directly.

Fung[7] pointed out that these two models are actually the same and with a proper definition of the elements can be converted from one to another. The same is true for the more complex analogies in Figure 2, which have more parameters but yield the same type of expression for the velocity of shortening. The only reason for preferring one model is the clarity of the physiological meaning of its parameters, and the possibility of carrying simple experiments to measure them. It is therefore appropriate to adopt Fung's suggestion of using the Maxwell body, and attribute this model to its originator A. V. Hill.[10]

5. Mathematical Description of Left Ventricle

The left ventricle is the essential part of the cardiac pump; it can be modeled in general as a pressure source. However, there is no agreement on the exact control of activity, or whether the left ventricle is a constant pressure or rather a constant volume flow. However, since it is easier and more convenient to work with pressure the numerous analytical models of the left ventricular function that have reported in the literature consider the ventricle as a pump for blood pressure. Nevertheless, they differ considerably in the geometric representation, the structure of the ventricular wall and the complexity of ventricular action. All the various models assume that the inner surface is loaded with stresses that result from and are equal to the left ventricular pressure, while the outer surfaces are relatively stress free. In contrast to skeletal muscle, the cardiac muscle will contract as a unit at the appearance of an excitation pulse, and there is no recruitment of motor unit according to required muscle activity. The pressure-volume relation in the ventricle is determined by the geometry and the distensibility of the cardiac muscle, and hence models that differ in one of these parameters will give different descriptions of the mechanics of ventricular function.

Three distinct muscle layers can be determined in the wall of the left ventricle. In this layer the muscle fibers spiral around the ventricular chamber at different major directions. Modeling these three layers is very complex and it is therefore easier to assume only two surfaces of revolution that represent the epicardial and endocardial surfaces, but even simpler models were suggested. In the past the muscle fibers were not considered in the ventricular model and the wall was viewed as a curved membrane with two principal radii of curvature. This assumption, even if the wall is considered to have a finite thickness with uniformly distributed muscle fibers, leads to the Laplace solution which appeared till now in the various physiology textbooks. The geometry of the vessel was approximated by a thin-walled ellipsoidal of rotation, thick-walled spheres, hollow cylinders, and ellipsoids. The ellipsoids are usually considered with their tops cut off, and with wall thicknesses that vary from the base of the left ventricle to the apex, being thinnest at the apex. The wall materials, in most models, are considered isotropic, with uniform circumferential stresses that relate to the pressure inside the chamber. These assumptions are used to simplify the the mathematical model.

The simplest assumption on the mechanism of pressure production inside the left ventricle was suggested by Wood[17] that adopted Laplace's derivation for the pressure difference across the wall of a curved volume of revolution and its relation to surface tension. In this model the relation between pressure difference and tension is given by the law of Laplace

$$P = T \left(\frac{1}{R_1} + \frac{1}{R_2} \right) \tag{17}$$

where T is the tension in the wall and R_1 and R_2 are the principal radii of curvature at any point of the ventricular wall. This assumes that the ventricular wall behaves as a membrane, although Wood showed that because of differences in the radii of curvature the pressure near the apex, for example, is much higher than at other locations on the ventricular wall and therefore there is an associated difference in vessel thickness.

The use of thin-walled models and especially the simple form of Laplace's Law is not justifiable for the left ventricle where the thickness of the vessel's wall is not very small compared with the radius of curvature. It is therefore necessary to develop an appropriate model for a thick-wall elastic chamber. For such a model a thick ellipsoidal shell can be considered, as shown in Figure 4, with symmetry, so that the shear stresses and the bending moments can be neglected. The myocardium is assumed as isotropic and homogeneous elastic material that obey Hookes' law. This law assumes that all deformations are in the elastic domain, and there is a linear relation between the strain and stress tensors, given by the following relation:

$$\epsilon_{ij} = \frac{1+\nu}{E} \sigma_{ij} - \frac{\nu}{E} \sigma_{ii} \delta_{ij} \tag{18}$$

where σ_{ij} and ϵ_{ij} are stress and strain tensors, E Youngs' modulus and ν Poisson's ratio. Since the myocardium behaves like an incompressible material it is justifiable to simplify the mathematics by taking the Poisson's ratio to be equal to one half. Thus, Equation 18 can be written in a simpler way. The expression for the strain tensor can be further simplified by the fact that the myocardium undergoes only radial distortion, along the radius of curvature, and the inertia forces of the cardiac muscles are negligible. The strains are related to the radius of curvature of the ventricle. Following the procedure suggested by Wong and Rautaharju[18] the two radii of curvature are related to each other by the following relation

$$r = (1 + \lambda \sin^2 \phi) R = kR \tag{19}$$

where ϕ is the angle between the semimajor axis and the radius of curvature, shown in Figure 5, and λ is a parameter, which is equal to 1 for a paraboloid, $\lambda = 0$ for a sphere and $\lambda > -1$ for ellipsoid. Hence, for the left ventricle this constant will be taken as $-1 < \lambda < 0$.

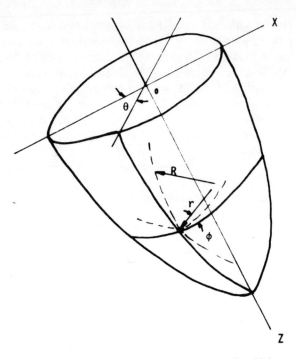

FIGURE 4.   Geometric description of the ellipsoidal assumption of the left ventricle and the two radii of curvature, r and R.

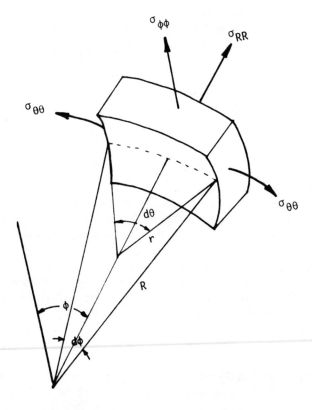

FIGURE 5.   The relation between the two radii of curvature
in a shell element cut from the left ventricular wall.

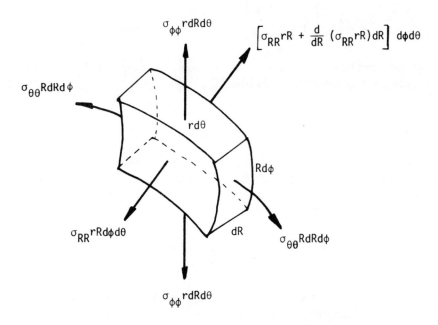

FIGURE 6.   Stress equilibrium in a shell element cut from the left ventricular wall.

With these assumptions Equation 18 can be written as follows:

$$E \frac{dU}{dR} = \sigma_{RR} - \tfrac{1}{2}(\sigma_{\theta\theta} + \sigma_{\phi\phi})$$

$$E \frac{U}{r} = \sigma_{\theta\theta} - \tfrac{1}{2}(\sigma_{RR} + \sigma_{\phi\phi}) \qquad (20)$$

$$E \frac{U}{R} = \sigma_{\phi\phi} - \tfrac{1}{2}(\sigma_{RR} + \sigma_{\theta\theta})$$

where U is the radial displacement of the myocardium.

Since the strains are functions of the radii of curvatures only, k in Equation 19 can be considered as a constant. Again following the Wong and Rautaharju[18] derivation, the longitudinal and latitudinal forces acting on a volume element, shown in Figure 6, cancel each other and only the radial forces are in equilibrium, thus they must satisfy the following relation:

$$2\sigma_{\phi\phi}\cdot rdRd\theta \sin \frac{d\phi}{2} + 2\sigma_{\theta\theta}\cdot Rd\phi dR \sin \frac{d\theta}{2}$$

$$= \frac{d}{dR}(R\cdot r\cdot\sigma_{RR})dR\, d\theta\, d\phi \qquad (21)$$

which for small angles $(d\theta, d\phi)$ is reduced to

$$\frac{d}{dR}(\sigma_{RR}\, rR) - R\,\sigma_{\theta\theta} - r\sigma_{\phi\phi} = 0 \qquad (22)$$

Equation 20 gives a differential equation for the radial displacement U:

$$\frac{dU}{dR} + \left(1 + \frac{1}{k}\right) \frac{U}{R} = 0 \tag{23}$$

This equation can be obtained explicitly only due to assumption of incompressibility. The solution to this equation is given by

$$U = Uo\, R^{-\frac{k+1}{k}} \tag{24}$$

where Uo is a constant that is to be determined by the pressures acting on the vessel walls. It is possible now to express, from Equation 19, the stresses $\sigma_{\bullet\bullet}$ and $\sigma_{\bullet\bullet}$ in terms of σ_{RR} and $U(R)$. Doing so and inserting these expressions into Equation 22, results in a differential equation for σ_{RR}, in the form:

$$R^2 \frac{d\sigma_{RR}}{dR} + \frac{k+1}{k} R\sigma_{RR} = \frac{4E}{3}\left(\frac{k^2 + k + 1}{k^2}\right) Uo\, R^{-\left(\frac{k+1}{k}\right)} \tag{25}$$

Solving this equation and calculating the longitudinal and latitudinal stresses from Equation 20, gives the following relations

$$\sigma_{RR} = A\, R^{-\left(\frac{k-1}{k}\right)} - \frac{4E}{3}\, Uo\, \frac{k^2 + k + 1}{k(k+2)}\, R^{-\left(\frac{2k+1}{k}\right)}$$

$$\sigma_{\theta\theta} = A\, R^{-\left(\frac{k-1}{k}\right)} - \frac{2E}{3}\, Uo\, \frac{k^2 - 2k - 2}{k(k+2)}\, R^{-\left(\frac{2k+1}{k}\right)} \tag{26}$$

$$\sigma_{\phi\phi} = A\, R^{-\left(\frac{k+1}{k}\right)} + 2E\, Uo\, \frac{1}{k+2}\, R^{-\left(\frac{2k+1}{k}\right)}$$

where A and Uo are constants that must be determined from the boundary conditions. The boundary conditions are given on both sides of the cardiac muscle. The outer surface of the cardiac muscle is exposed to intrathoracic pressure which is very small in comparison to the inner pressure, which is the intraventricular pressure. Thus, the boundary conditions can be taken as

$$\sigma_{RR} = Po \;@\; R = Ro$$

$$\sigma_{RR} = 0 \;@\; R = Ro + To \tag{27}$$

where Ro and To are radius of curvature and wall thickness at a particular location, chosen here at the vortex of the shell, namely $\phi = 0$. This gives the final form of the stresses within the cardiac muscle

$$\sigma_{RR} = \frac{Po}{To}\left\{ Ro + To - R\right\}\left(\frac{Ro}{R}\right)^{\frac{2k+1}{k}}$$

$$\sigma_{\theta\theta} = \frac{Po}{To}\left\{\left(\frac{Ro + To}{2}\right)\frac{k^2 - 2k - 2}{k^2 + k + 1} - R\right\}\left(\frac{Ro}{R}\right)^{\frac{2k+1}{k}} \tag{28}$$

$$\sigma_{\phi\phi} = \frac{Po}{To}\left\{\frac{3}{2}(Ro + To)\frac{k}{k^2 + k + 1} + R\right\}\left(\frac{Ro}{R}\right)^{\frac{2k+1}{k}}$$

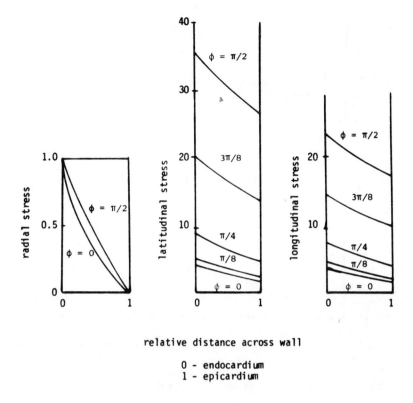

FIGURE 7.   Stress-distribution in vessel wall, normalized in relation to P_o.

The equations are written for a specified value of ϕ, and the radius of curvature and wall thickness varies with this angle, with $\phi = 0$ corresponds to the apex and $\phi = \pi/2$ to the base of the ellipsoid.

These equations can be used to calculate the distribution of stresses across the vessel wall, from endocardium to epicardium. The results for a ventricle with volume of 200 cc, correspond to $Ro = 1.8$ cm at the apex, and uniform wall thickness of 0.8 cm are shown in Figure 7. It is noted that the longitudinal and latitudinal stresses are relatively uniform near the apex and vary nearly linearly near the base of the ventricle, and both are much larger than the radial component. The absolute value of these stresses decreases with an increase in wall thickness. It looks, at first, as a better arrangement, however, a small increase in wall thickness increases the mass of the left ventricle, and hence, the required energy for maintenance and contraction, and thus decreases significantly the cardiac pump efficiency. The amount of change in longitudinal and latitudinal stresses as a function of increased wall thickness is shown in Figure 8. It should be noted that the changes between the longitudinal and latitudinal stresses are due to the geometry of the ventricle, and are equal for the limiting case of spherical geometry.

Another possible model was suggested by Talbot and Gessner.[16] They considered a hollow cylinder, with circumferentially arranged fibers. The cylinder is closed at both ends, thus having a uniform axial stress that must balance the pressure acting on these ends. This uniform axial stress also results in a uniform constant axial strain, K. Equation 20 can be written for this case as follows:

$$E \frac{du}{dr} = \sigma_{rr} - \frac{1}{2}(\sigma_t + \sigma_z)$$

$$E \frac{u}{r} = \sigma_t - \frac{1}{2}(\sigma_{rr} + \sigma_z) \qquad (29)$$

$$EK = \sigma_z - \frac{1}{2}(\sigma_{rr} + \sigma_z)$$

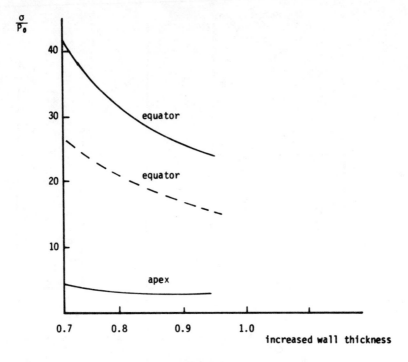

FIGURE 8.   The amount of change in longitudinal (broken line) and latitudinal (solid line) stresses as a function of increased wall thickness.

where σ_t is the tangential stress, σ_z is the axial stress, and σ_{rr} and u are the radial stress and displacement, respectively. Again, as in the previous model, it is possible to assume a general Poisson's ratio, as in Talbot and Gessner, it is, however, easier to assume incompressibility and to take $\nu = \frac{1}{2}$. For this case the following equation for the radial displacement is obtained

$$\frac{du}{dr} + \frac{u}{r} + K = 0 \qquad\qquad (30)$$

whose solution is given by

$$u = \frac{A}{r} - \frac{k}{2} r \qquad\qquad (31)$$

where A is a constant to be determined from the boundary conditions.

Inserting this expression into Equation 28 and solving for the stresses, yields

$$\sigma_{rr} = -\frac{2}{3} \frac{A}{r^2} - K + \sigma_z$$

$$\qquad\qquad (32)$$

$$\sigma_t = \frac{2}{3} \frac{A}{r^2} - K + \sigma_z$$

It is obvious from the last two equations that the uniform axial stress can be incorporated into the constant, and evaluated in the same way from the boundary condition. These conditions are the same as for the last model, namely, the inner radial stress must equal the intraventricular pressure, while the outer radial stress is taken as zero, thus neglecting the intrathoracic pressure. This gives

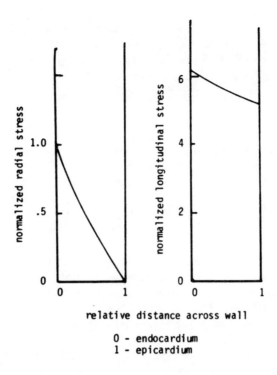

FIGURE 9.   Stress distribution in the vessel wall for cylindrical ventricle.

$$\sigma_{rr} = \frac{Ro^2}{To^2 + 2RoTo} \left[\left(\frac{Ro + To}{r} \right)^2 - 1 \right] Po$$

$$\sigma_t = -\frac{Ro^2}{To^2 + 2RoTo} \left[1 + \left(\frac{Ro + To}{r} \right)^2 \right] Po$$

(33)

where Ro is the inside diameter of the assumed ventricular cylinder and To is the vessel thickness, and Po is the intraventricular pressure. The axial stress is given by

$$\sigma_z = \frac{Po}{\left(\frac{Ro + To}{Ro} \right)^2 - 1} = \frac{Ro^2}{To^2 + 2RoTo} Po$$

(34)

Comparing this model with the ellipsoidal model, reveals that the shape of the pressures within the vessel wall, Figure 9, are actually the same. However, the level of stresses is much smaller in the cylindrical case, and the average stress, calculated per unit wall thickness, is reduced to the simple Laplace's relation.

The relation used for the last model assumes a specific value for Ro and To, this is true for any instant, but it varies during the cardiac cycle. If these quantities are used to describe the end diastolic radius and wall thickness, the appropriate parameters, R and T, are given by the conservation of mass as:

$$(R + T)^2 - R^2 = (Ro + To)^2 - Ro^2 = \text{constant}$$

(35)

This permits the evaluation of stresses in the ventricular wall as a function of the ventricular volume, if the dependence of internal radius on time is known. Assuming average quantities this can be related to fiber force, Talbot and Gessner.[16]

This, however, requires the knowledge of the fiber cross section and its unstressed conditions. An example of such analysis is given by Beneken and DeWitt.[4]

6. Flow Through Heart Valves

The main pump of the heart, which transfers oxygenated blood from the lungs to the systemic circulation, has two nonreturn valves: the mitral valve between the left atrium (the collecting chamber) and the left ventricle (the pumping chamber), and the aortic valve between the left ventricle and the aortic arch. In both valves the normal operation depends on the valve structure and the geometry of the valve housing (adjacent geometry).

The aortic valve of a human consists of three nonmuscular cusps (flaps, leaflets) of approximately the same crescent-shaped geometry and only 0.1-0.4 mm thick. In the filling stage (diastole) these three leaflets are closed against each other to prevent backflow into the heart. During the ejection period the cusps fold back toward the aorta to permit the blood to flow into the aortic arch. Because of the semilunar shape they attain during diastole, the valve is also called the semilunar valve. Although the leaflets are extremely thin with very small mass they have different compositions of tissue on its two surfaces. The face toward the aorta is composed of highly densed interlacing collagen fibers, with reinforcement in the area of maximum stress, while the opposite surface is composed of a soft layer of spongy connective tissue.

In the aorta there is a permanent marked dilatation, corresponding to each of the cusps. These dilatations of the aorta are called sinuses, and from them branch the two coronary arteries (ostia) which supply the cardiac muscle with fresh oxygenated blood.

The inlet valve, situated between the left atrial and left ventricular chambers and called the mitral valve, consists of two valve leaflets attached around the mitral orifice perimeter by an atrio-ventricular fibrous ring. The two leaflets are not of the size, and the larger anterior leaflet opens a great distance more than the smaller posterior one. As the pressure difference across the mitral valve is much smaller than that of the aortic valve, the cusps are with less collageneous fibers, and consist of only a thin endocardial lining which offers very little resistance to blood flow. The mitral valve is open to its maximum during the rapid filling stage, and closes partially during the slow filling. At the end of the diastole the valve closes, to prevent retrograded flow back into the atrium during the short period of isometric contraction. The two cusps of the mitral valve are not controlled by the blood flow, as is the case with the aortic valve, but also by the contraction mechanism of the left ventricle. The margins of the two cusps are connected to the papillary muscle on the opposite wall, near the apex, by the chordae tendineae. Thus the contraction of the heart causes geometric changes in the operation of the valves, which also prevents the prolapse of the valve.

The function of the sinuses in the normal operation of the aortic valve has been a subject of speculation from as early as the sixteenth century, when Leonardo da Vinci in 1513 suggested the theory that the aortic dilatation behind the valves would produce a vortex, which must be essential to the control mechanism of aortic flow. More than 200 years later Valsalva in 1740 speculated that the sinuses are important to the dissipation of the violence of systolic contraction. There were many experiments to justify and to resist these theories, as well as newer theories. As the following discussion will show there is some truth in these theories, however, the functions assigned to the sinuses are incorrectly stated.

7. Flow in the Aortic Valve

According to Bellhouse and Talbot[3] there are four marked phases in the cycle of the aortic valve:

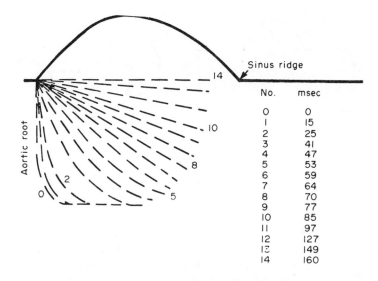

No.	msec
0	0
1	15
2	25
3	41
4	47
5	53
6	59
7	64
8	70
9	77
10	85
11	97
12	127
13	149
14	160

FIGURE 10. Position of leaflet and time reference in aortic valve motion. (From Hung, T. K. and Schuessler, G. V., *J. Biomech.*, 10, 597, 1977. With permission.)

Opening Phase — In this phase there is a yield to pressure differences across the valve by forward motion of the valve leaflets without opening of the valve and, hence, with no flow. This period, which is very short and lasts about 50 milliseconds, is followed by an equal duration when the valve starts from the shut to the fully open position.

Stationary Phase — The leaflets are stationary in the fully open position, thus allowing blood to flow from the left ventricle into the aorta.

Deceleration Phase — At the stationary phase when the leaflets are fully open the formation of vortex inside the cusps causes an increase in pressure on the outer surface of the cusps, causing them to move into the flowing blood toward closure.

Reversed Flow — After the cusps have moved slightly from the fully open position a small amount of reversed flow, caused by waves reflected from the carotid branch, is pushing the valve till it is completely sealed. In this period there is a retrograded flow into the left ventricle, that might amount, in a normal human, to 5% of the forward flow. In diseased valves it might even reach higher values.

The complexity of flow conditions and the nonlinear characteristics of the flow and cusp motion in the opening phase make the problem intractable analytically. However, simplified solutions for pressure and flow at different phases were published in the last decade. These solutions explain part of the valve characteristics and of the control mechanism. Only a few of these solutions were actually tested experimentally, and most of them refer to the excellent experiments carried out by Bellhouse and Bellhouse[2] and Bellhouse.[1]

In the opening phase the cusps are shut and pressure is being built up against them inside the left ventricle. In response to this pressure they bulge forward and then rapidly open and move forward with no resistance to flow. The shape of the leaflets in this forward motion are very difficult to obtain, since measurements in such a rapid transient flow are very complex. Hung and Schuessler[11] assumed a reference for such leaflet motion, Figure 10, and solved with the finite-difference method the effects of such shapes variations on the flow.

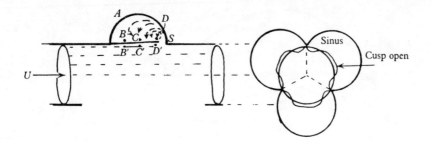

FIGURE 11.   Streamlines for steady flow through the aortic valve. (From Bellhouse, B. and Talbot, L., *Circ. Res.*, 25, 693, 1969. With permission.)

After the leaflets reach the fully open position they remain fully open during the stationary phase, which occupies about 55% of the systole. For the forward motion through the valve the flow can be considered steady, although within the sinus ridge there is a slow buildup of pressure in preparation for the closure of the leaflets in the next stage. The geometry for the quasisteady flow is given in Figure 11.

The flow through the valve can be considered a steady flow. Inside the cusps there is a formation of vortex that was observed by Bellhouse and Talbot.[3] They suggested to model the sinus vortex by one half of the Hill spherical vortex. This is a model of vortices that neglects the viscous effect of the flow and results in vortex formation inside a sphere. For such a flow there is a stream function, Ψ, given by

$$\Psi = - \frac{A}{10} (a^2 - r^2) \, r^2 \sin^2 \theta \tag{36}$$

where A is a constant, and r, θ are defined in Figure 12. The associated velocities are

$$r = - \frac{1}{r^2 \sin \theta} \frac{\partial \Psi}{\partial \theta} = \frac{A}{5} (a^2 - r^2) \cos \theta$$

$$\theta = \frac{1}{r \sin \theta} \frac{\partial \Psi}{\partial r} = - \frac{A}{5} (A^2 - 2r^2) \sin \theta \tag{37}$$

where the flow is assumed steady.

The pressure, for this case of steady flow is given by the computation of the total head; H, according to

$$H = \frac{p}{\rho} + \frac{1}{2} \left| \, v \, \right|^2$$

$$\vec{\nabla} H = \vec{v} \times \text{curl } \vec{v} \tag{38}$$

which gives

$$\frac{\partial H}{\partial r} = v_\theta - \left[\frac{\partial}{\partial r} (r v_\theta) - \frac{\partial v_r}{\partial \theta} \right] = - \frac{A^2}{5} r (a^2 - 2r^2) \sin^2 \theta$$

$$\frac{\partial H}{\partial \theta} = - r v_r \left[\frac{\partial}{\partial r} (r v_\theta) - \frac{\partial v_r}{\partial \theta} \right] = - \frac{A^2}{5} r^2 (a^2 - r^2) \sin \theta \cos \theta \tag{39}$$

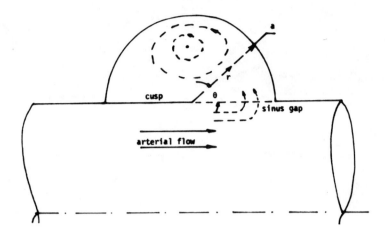

FIGURE 12.   Hill spherical vortex as a model of the flow inside the aortic sinus.

Integration of the last equation and using the boundary condition of stagnation pressure, Po, at the stagnation points $r = 0$, $\theta = 0$, π yield the total head

$$H = \frac{P}{\rho} + \frac{1}{2} [v]^2 = \frac{Po}{\rho} - \frac{A^2}{10} (a^2 r^2 - r^2) \sin^2 \theta \qquad (40)$$

Inserting the velocity given by Equation 37 into the last equation and using the total head of the aortic flow given by:

$$H_a = \frac{P_a}{\rho} + \frac{1}{2} U^2 = \frac{P_o}{\rho} \qquad (41)$$

where P_a is the aortic pressure, results in the following equation, which gives the sinus pressure by the aortic pressure at the valve entrance:

$$\frac{P - P_a}{\frac{1}{2}\rho U^2} = 1 - \frac{A^2 a^4}{50} \left\{ 1 - 2 \left(\frac{r}{a} \right)^2 + \left(\frac{r}{a} \right)^4 \right.$$
$$\left. + \sin^2 \theta \left[3 \left(\frac{r}{a} \right)^2 - 2 \left(\frac{r}{a} \right)^4 \right] \right\} \qquad (42)$$

Bellhouse and Talbot[3] showed that the vortex is generated by convective processes and to a much lesser extent by diffusive processes, thus assuming that the vorticity at the core of the sinus is proportional to the angular velocity of the inflow to the sinus. With these assumptions they wrote the constant A as

$$A = \frac{\sqrt{2} \alpha U}{a^2} \qquad (43)$$

where α is another constant.

By integrating Equation 42 over the cusp surface, and writing the average sinus pressure as $\overline{Ps}$, they obtained, for the special case when the cusp length is $3/2$ a, the following relation:

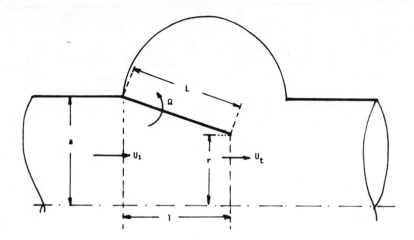

FIGURE 13.   Schematic diagram of pulsatile flow through the aortic valve.

$$\frac{\overline{Ps} - Pa}{\frac{1}{2}\rho U^2} = 1 - 0.0672 \, \alpha^2 \qquad (44)$$

By experiment they obtained the value of $\alpha = 3.21$, which in turn resulted in a peak velocity that equals 0.91U. Despite the fact that viscosity is neglected, that the cusps are taken as rigid and the sinus as a sphere, the results agree well with their experiments. A better analysis must consider the displacement of the vortex core toward the sinus ridge and might even lead to trailing vortexes, but will add considerably to the complexity of the problem, as pointed out by Bellhouse and Talbot.

This pressure difference is gradually pushing the valve to its closed position, which is the deceleration phase. The analysis of the flow of this phase was also given in their solution in the following way:

The cusps are assumed of length L, moving with an angular velocity Ω. The geometry and pressure at the planes of the aortic ring and the cusp tip are (a, P_1) and $(r, P_t,)$ respectively. The distance along the cusp is denoted by x and the cross-section radius is y, as described in Figure 13.

The conservation of mass within the control volume is given by

$$\pi \, a^2 \, U_1 \; - \; \pi \, r^2 \, U_t = \int_{(L)} \vec{v} \cdot \vec{ds} \qquad (45)$$

In their article they wrote the right-hand side of the equation as dv/dt, although their results are correct this should be written as $(\partial v / \partial \theta \cdot d\theta / dt)$, as the variation of volume with changes in cusp tip radius should not be included. The velocities U_1 and U_t are average velocities at the corresponded planes. This equation after integration yields the following relation for the velocities.

$$U_t = \frac{U_1}{\lambda^2} - \frac{\Omega a}{3\lambda^2} \left(\frac{L}{a}\right)^2 (1 + 2\lambda) \qquad (46)$$

where λ is the nondimensional parameter $\lambda = (r/a)$. The integration over the entire cusp, can be replaced by integration from the aortic ring to any cross-section, thus give

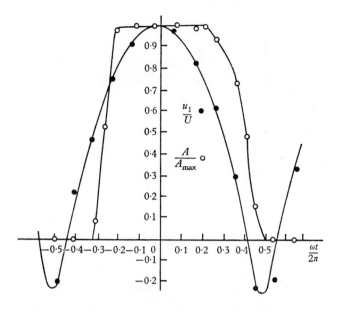

FIGURE 14. Aortic velocity and valve opening area as a function of time. (From Bellhouse, B. and Talbot, L., *Circ. Res.*, 25, 693, 1969. With permission.)

$$U(x, t) = \frac{a^2}{y^2} U_1 - \frac{a\Omega}{3} \left(\frac{x}{y}\right)^2 \left(1 + \frac{2y}{a}\right) \tag{47}$$

Since the pipe axis is a streamline, the average velocity can be inserted into the unsteady Bernoulli equation

$$\int_0^{\ell} \frac{\partial u}{\partial t} \, d\ell + \frac{1}{2} \left[U^2 \right]_0^{\ell} = -\frac{1}{\rho} (P_t - P_1) \tag{48}$$

where ℓ is the distance along the axis, given for the cusp tip by

$$\ell = \alpha \left[\left(\frac{L}{a}\right)^2 - (1 - \lambda)^2 \right]^{\frac{1}{2}} \tag{49}$$

carrying out the integration result in the following relation between the aortic ring and cusps tip pressure, in the following form:

$$\frac{P_1 - P_t}{\rho a} = \frac{\ell}{\lambda} \left[\frac{\partial U_1}{\partial t} - \frac{a}{3} \left(\frac{L}{a}\right)^2 \frac{d\Omega}{dt} \right] + \frac{1}{2a} \left(\frac{1}{\lambda^4} - 1\right) U_1{}^2$$

$$+ \frac{1}{18\lambda} \left(\frac{L}{a}\right)^4 (1 + 2\lambda)^2 \, a \, \Omega^2 \tag{50}$$

$$- \frac{1}{3\lambda^4} \left(\frac{L}{a}\right)^2 (1 + \lambda) \, \Omega \, U_1$$

Equations 50 and 46 enable the calculation of the tip velocity from the time-dependent velocity through the value $U_1(t)$, and the observed rate of cusp closure. For the data given in Figure 14 with $U = 71.2$ cm/sec Bellhouse and Talbot[3] obtained the pressure difference described in Figure 15.

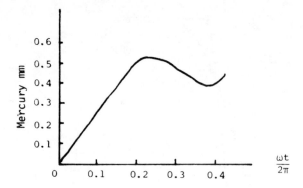

FIGURE 15.   Calculated average pressure across the valve during valve closure. (From Bellhouse, B. and Talbot, L., *Circ. Res.*, 25, 693, 1969. With permission.)

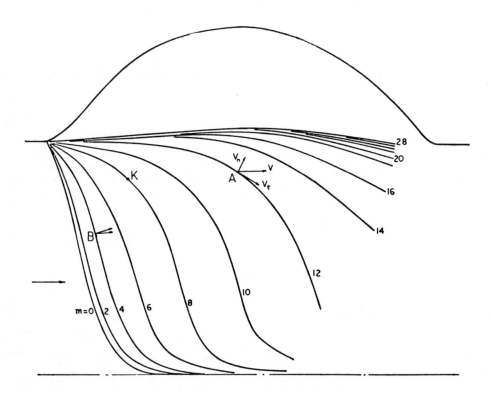

FIGURE 16.   Positions of leaflet in valve motion shown at 28 intervals. K-point of maximum curvature and hence maximum bending stress. (From Swanson, W. and Clark, R. E., *Circ. Res.*, 32, 42, 1973. With permission.)

These flow conditions will persist until a reflected pressure wave is strong enough to push the cusp into its closed position. This period of reversed flow is highly complex and depends very strongly on the cusp's elastic coefficients and the geometric and histological condition of the aortic arch and the carotid branches. It is highly complex, mathematically, and needs not only more sophisticated analysis which is very difficult, but requires considering the exact shape of the cusp and its exact location at the time of arrival of the reversed flow.

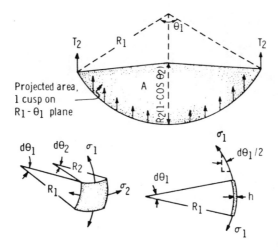

FIGURE 17. Balance of forces in a leaflet element. (From Chong et al., *Biomater. Med. Devices Artif. Organs*, 1, 307, 1973. With permission.)

Attempts to obtain the exact cusp position during systole were made by many investigators, as for example, Swanson and Clark[14,15] who assumed time averaged flow rates and obtained leaflet positions as a function of pressure and time, as described in Figure 16.

8. Stresses in the Aortic Valve

The stresses within the aortic valve leaflets are very difficult to obtain by direct measurements, because of their very thin structure. It is more appropriate in this case to obtain the stress, or even the order of magnitude of these stresses by analytical consideration. For this purpose the leaflets can be considered as thin membrane with two principal radii of curvature, with negligible or very small mass. The interesting period, from stresses point of view, is the diastole, when the leaflets are subjected to maximum loads.

Taking an element of the leaflet, Figure 17, and writing the balance of forces in the normal and axial component, the following equations are obtained; Chong et al.[5]

$$2\left(h\,\sigma_1\,\frac{d\theta_1}{2}\right)R_2 d\theta_2 \; + \; 2\left(h\,\sigma_2\,\frac{d\theta_2}{2}\right)R_1 d\theta_1$$
$$= R(R_1 d\theta_1)(R_2 d\theta_2) \tag{51}$$

$$P\left\{\frac{\theta_1}{2}R_1^2 \; - \; [R_1 - R_2(1-\cos\theta_2)]\,R_1\,\sin\frac{\theta_1}{2}\right\}$$
$$= T_2 R_1 \theta_1 \tag{52}$$

where R_1 and R_2 are the two principal radii of curvature, σ_1 and σ_2 are the principal stresses, h is the thickness of the aortic leaflet, P is the pressure difference across the membrane and θ_1 and θ_2 are the subtending angles.

By introducing $T_1 = \sigma_1 h$ and $T_2 = \sigma_2 h$, Equation 51 is reduced to the simple Laplace equation:

$$\frac{T_1}{R_1} + \frac{T_2}{R_2} = P \tag{53}$$

Thus, giving the tensile forces in the aortic leaflets as:

$$T_1 = \frac{PR_1}{2} \left\{ 2 - \frac{R_1}{R_2} + \frac{R_1}{R_2} \left[1 - \frac{R_2}{R_1} (1 - \cos \theta_2) \right] \frac{\sin \theta_{1/2}}{\theta_{1/2}} \right\}$$

$$T_2 = \frac{PR_1}{2} \left\{ 1 - \left[1 - \frac{R_2}{R_1} (1 - \cos \theta_2) \right] \frac{\sin \theta_{1/2}}{\theta_{1/2}} \right\}$$

(54)

or in nondimensional form

$$\frac{T_1}{PR_1} = 1 - \frac{1}{2} f(\theta_1)(1 - \cos \theta_2) - \frac{1}{2} \lambda \left[1 - f(\theta_1) \right]$$

(55)

$$\frac{T_2}{PR_2} = \frac{\lambda}{2} \left[1 - f(\theta_1) \right] + f(\theta_1)(1 - \cos \theta_2)$$

where

$$f(\theta_1) = \frac{\sin \theta_{1/2}}{\theta_{1/2}} \; ; \; \lambda = \frac{R_1}{R_2}$$

From these equations it is clear that T_1 has a minimum, where T_2 has a maximum at $\cos \theta_2 = 1$, or $\theta_2 = 180°$. Thus having the force in the axial direction predominant for this valve geometry.

The same approach is too complex for different configurations as for example the case where the cusps are assumed to be ellipsoid of revolution. For such cases it is more convenient to use the general equilibrium equation for thin shells in the form of surface of revolution, with negligible bending, i.e., obeying the membrane shell theory. For this case the equations are given by Timoshenko and Woinowsky-Kriger[19] as:

$$\frac{\partial}{\partial \phi} (R_0 N_\phi) + \frac{\partial N \theta \phi}{\partial \theta} R_1 - N\theta R_1 \cos \phi + F_y' \cdot R_1 R_0 = 0$$

$$\frac{\partial}{\partial \phi} (R_0 N_\phi \theta) + \frac{\partial N\theta}{\partial \theta} R_1 + N\theta\phi R_1 \cos \phi + F_x' R_1 R_0 = 0 \quad (56)$$

$$\frac{N\phi}{R_1} + \frac{N\theta}{R_2} = - F_z'$$

where $N\phi$ and $N\theta$ are the normal forces per unit length, where ϕ (θ_1 in the previous analysis) and θ (θ_2 in the previous analysis) are measured from a specific location on the meridian plane. F_x, F_y, and F_z are the intensities of the external forces acting on the meridian plane. R_1 is the principal radius of curvature in the meridian plane and R_2 is the principal radius of curvature in the plane perpendicular to the meridian. R_0 is given by

$$R_0 = R_2 \sin \phi$$

(57)

Writing Equation 56 for the case of negligible shear stresses yields:

$$\frac{\partial}{\partial \phi} (r_0 N\phi) - N\theta \, r_1 \cos \phi = 0$$

$$\frac{\partial N\theta}{\partial \theta} = 0 \tag{58}$$

$$N_0 = P\star R_2 - N\phi \, \frac{R_2}{R_1}$$

where P* is the force that results from the internal pressure.

The solution to this set of equations is given by:

$$N = \frac{1}{R_0 \sin \phi} \int_0^\phi P\star R_1 R_2 \sin \Psi \cos \Psi \, d \Psi$$

$$= \frac{1}{R_0 \sin \phi} \int_0^\phi P\star R_1 R_0 \cos \Psi \, d \Psi \tag{59}$$

$$N\theta = P R_2 - \frac{R_2}{R_0 R_1 \sin \phi} \int_0^\phi P\star R_1 R_0 \cos \Psi \, d \Psi \tag{60}$$

For the special case where P* can be described by the product of the internal pressure and the projected area $P\star = P \pi R_0^2$ the equation can be simplified. In this case the first equation in Equation 58 can be written for a portion of the shell instead of an element, as described in Figure 18, thus giving

$$2 \pi R_0 N\phi \sin \phi - P\star = 0$$

or $\tag{61}$

$$N\phi = \frac{PR_0}{2 \sin \phi} = \frac{PR_2}{2}$$

which gives upon insertion into the third part of Equation 58:

$$N\theta = P \left(R_2 - \frac{R_2^2}{2R_1} \right) \tag{62}$$

For the special case of a sphere these equations give

$$N\phi = N\theta = \frac{PR}{2}$$

where $R = R_1 = R_2$.

In the case of a shell in the form of an ellipsoidal of revolution, with 2a and 2b as the major and the minor axes, where

$$R_1 = \frac{a^2 b^2}{(a^2 \sin^2 \phi + b^2 \cos^2 \phi)^{3/2}}$$

$$\tag{63}$$

$$R_2 = \frac{a^2}{(a^2 \sin^2 \phi + b^2 \cos^2 \phi)^{1/2}}$$

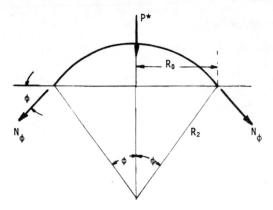

FIGURE 18.   Simplified geometry for shell deformation without bending.

the equations are reduced to:

$$N\phi = N\theta = \frac{Pa^2}{2b} \text{ at the top of the shell}$$

$$N\phi = \frac{Pa^2}{2} \quad N\theta = Pa\left(1 - \frac{a^2}{2b^2}\right) \text{ at the equator}$$

This shows that for this particular case $N\phi$ is always positive, while $N\theta$ might change sign if $a^2 > 2b^2$. From measurements of average radius of curvature carried out by Chong et al.[5] it can be seen that this is sometimes possible as a^2 and $2b^2$ are very close, which might lead to region with $N\theta = 0$, or even with stresses in opposite directions. This points out the importance of knowing the exact curvatures, especially in the design of artificial heart valves, which are not included in this text.

REFERENCES

1. Bellhouse, B. J., Velocity and pressure distribution in the aortic valve, *J. Fluid Mech.*, 37, 587, 1969.
2. Bellhouse, B. J. and Bellhouse, F., Fluid mechanics of model normal and stenosed aortic valve, *Circ. Res.*, 25, 693, 1969.
3. Bellhouse, B. J. and Talbot, L., The fluid mechanics of the aortic valve, *J. Fluid Mech.*, 35, 721, 1969.
4. Beneken, J. E. W. and DeWitt, B., A physical approach to hemodynamic aspects of the human cardiovascular system, in *Physical Bases of Circulatory Transport*, Reeve, E. B. and Guyton, A. C., Eds., W. B. Saunders, Philadelphia, 1967, 1.
5. Chong, K. P., Wieting, D. W., Hwang, N. H. C., and Kennedy, J. H., Stress analysis of normal human aortic valve leaflets during diastole, *Biomater. Med. Devices Artif. Organs*, 1, 307, 1973.
6. Fung, V. C., A necessary modification of Hill's equation for cardiac muscle, *Fed. Proc.*, 29 (Abstr.), 839, 1970.
7. Fung, V. C., Comparison of different models of the heart muscle, *J. Biomech.*, 4, 289, 1971.
8. Hefner, L. L. and Brown, T. E., Elastic components of cat papillary muscle, *Am. J. Physiol.*, 212, 1221, 1967.
9. Hill, A. V., Heat of shortening and the dynamic constant of muscles, *Proc. R. Soc. London, Ser. B,* 126, 136, 1938.

10. Hill, A. V., Mechanics of the contractile element of muscle, *Nature (London),* 166, 415, 1950.
11. Hung, T. K. and Schuessler, G. V., An analysis of the hemodynamics of the opening of aortic valve, *J. Biomech.,* 10, 597, 1977.
12. Pollack, G. H., Maximum velocity as an index of contractility in cardiac muscle: A critical evaluation, *Circ. Res.,* 26, 111, 1970.
13. Sonnenblick, E. H., Force-velocity relations in mammalian heart muscle, *Am. J. Physiol.,* 202, 931, 1963.
14. Swanson, W. and Clark, R. E., Aortic valve leaflet motion during systole, *Circ. Res.,* 32, 42, 1973.
15. Swanson, W. and Clark, R. E., Dimensions and geometric relationship of the human aortic valve as a function of pressure, *Circ. Res.,* 35, 871, 1974.
16. Talbot, S. A. and Gessner, U., *System Physiology,* John Wiley & Sons, New York, 1973.
17. Wood, R. H., A few applications of a physical theorem to membranes in the human body in a state of tension, *J. Anat. Physiol.,* 26, 302, 1892.
18. Wong, A. V. K. and Rauthaharja, P. M., Stress distribution within the left ventricular wall approximated as a thick ellipsoidal shell, *Am. Heart J.,* 75, 649, 1968.
19. Timoshenko, P. and Woinowsky-Krieger, S., *Theory of Plates and Shells,* 2nd ed., McGraw-Hill, New York, 1959.

Chapter 9

BLOOD FLOW IN THE MICROCIRCULATION

A. Introduction

The term microcirculation refers to the flow of blood in small vessels. As simple as this definition sounds, it is very complex and periodically debatable, since the exact site of zone where blood vessels are defined as microcirculation varies from one textbook to another. They can be determined by their structure, as true capillaries consist of a thin tube of endothelial cells, and no connective tissue or smooth muscle. This enables the transcapillary exchange of the various substances but eliminates the possibility of active control. Another definition of the microcirculation is the circulation segment downstream of the precapillary sphincter, which is a zone reach with smooth muscle that controls the capillary wall in the terminal microvasculature.

From the dynamics of flow in these vessels the microcirculation is defined as the site where the flow can no longer be approximated by laminar flow since the vessel diameter is only a few times more than the actual size of the red blood cells, and the flow must be considered as multiphase flow with the red blood cells flowing in a single file formation and usually in a deformed state.

The vessels, in all of these definitions, range from about 4 μm to 20 μm in diameter and are about 0.04 to 0.05 mm in length. It is therefore clear that the red blood cells fold and bend as they pass through the microcirculation. Because of this deformation the red cells travel in a single file formation with bolus flow of plasma between them. It is important to note that the number of cells passing with a specific volume might vary from one capillary to another. For unknown reasons, some capillaries are filled with red cells at certain instances, while others at the same instance carry very few or even no red cells. Not only is the number of cells passing through a capillary constantly shifting, but so is the population of active and inactive capillaries. The amount of blood delivered to the capillaries is controlled by shunts between the arterial and venous sides of the microcirculation via the Arterio-Venous-Anastomosis (AVA) whose diameter can vary. The diameter of the AVA and the activity of the neighboring microcirculatory bed determines whether a particular capillary is active or inactive. This adds to a phenomenon found by Nichol et al.[43] and Burton[8] and known as the critical closure. Burton and Yamada[9] found that when the transmural pressure is reduced to a certain low level (the critical closure pressure) the flow is abruptly ceased. This phenomenon is known to exist in cases of ischemia in various muscles or in the legs with phegmasia cerulea dolens. However, Burton's explanation that relates this closure to active tension in the capillary wall, which is based on Laplace's law, is too simple and can lead to errors, as pointed out by Azuma and Oka.[4] They showed that the elastic elements under normal physiological conditions are under compression and there is no elastic tension activity to constrict the vessels, thus contradicts the whole basis of Burton's theory.

As the essential function of the capillaries is the supply of all the nutritional requirements of various organs and tissues, and since different organs require different amounts of nutrition, the amount of capillaries in them is different. This leads to a different number of capillaries in 1 mm^2 of tissue (capillary count). Not only is the number of capillaries different, but also the structure, permeability, and other parameters, which vary from one organ to another.

Because of their small size and large number, the capillaries have a very large surface to volume ratio thus achieving a much higher exposure of the species to the exchange surface. This exchange of material across the capillary wall is accomplished by convective and diffusive processes governed mainly by the interstitial fluid concentration.

There is also back and forth shifting of plasma water from and to the interstitial fluids. This is known as ultrafiltration, which must be a function of the rate at which a given substance is used or produced by flowing blood and tissue cells.

The permeability of the capillary wall must be considered with conjunction to particular substances, as different substances "pass" the capillary wall by different mechanisms and at different rates. Not all the transport mechanisms are completely understood. The blood cells, bacteria and plasma proteins can "pass" through the intracellular cement by diffusion, while other substances such as water, glucose, urea, and various electrolytes can diffuse also through the endothelial lining. The average size of pores in the endothelial layer is 30 to 40 Å, however, it is estimated that there are pores with much higher diameter (250 to 350 Å) with a very low frequency. Charm and Kurland[11] estimated that there is one large pore for every 34,000 small pores. The porosity of the endothelial layer together with the diffusion properties of the elements determines the fluid exchange. The differences in chemical potential which actually control the diffusion are not known, and are usually replaced by the differences between ambient hydrostatic pressures and the colloid osmotic pressure on both sides of the wall, which leads to Starling's hypothesis, which will be discussed in the text.

The average velocity of blood flow in the capillary is 0.07 cm/sec, and with an average length of 0.04 to 0.05 mm, the average transit time for blood is less than one second.

B. Elasticity of Red Blood Cell

The geometry of the red blood cell was described in Chapter 3, and the average dimensions are given in Figure 1 of that chapter. Although there is a general agreement about these average dimensions, there is a wide spectrum of theories on the reason for this shape, the mechanical nature of its various components, and the shape which the red blood cell takes up when passing through the narrow vessels of the microcirculation, especially when the flow is halted and started again.

The simplest description of the red blood cell is that of a flexible membrane enclosing a viscoelastic incompressible material reach in hemoglobin. The interior of the cell can be described as a liquid, or as a solid gel. However, the hemoglobin molecule can become crystalized and behave like a solid, a situation known as sickle cell. This is not only a structural problem, but the exact definition of the cell's interior defines the mechanical behavior of the cell as it passes through the microvasculatory bed. The content of the interior forces the red blood cell to behave as an isochoric material (to deform without a change of volume), and in fact this is known to be the case.[50] In addition to nearly constant volume the surface area of the red blood cell membrane is nearly constant, even in very large extensions and severe deformations. Evans et al.[17] pointed out that the maximum dilatation of the membrane surface area prior to rupture is only 3 to 4%. If the interior is taken to be viscous liquid it can not resist a shear stress without flow[19]; this leads to a conclusion that the predominate factor in the stress-carrying mechanism is the mechanical parameter of the membrane and not the structure. On the other hand, if the interior is taken as a solid or a solid gel the mechanical behavior of the red blood cell is reduced to that of a deformable elastic body in flowing liquid and the deformations are obtained through calculation of finite-elasticity. Although the elastic, or viscoelastic, properties of the red cell are not well established there is a general agreement that the shape is determined by the elastic properties of its membrane, the assumption on its interior and the blood vessel in which it flows. The latter is even more important when the red blood cell penetrates through openings in the endothelial wall, which are only 0.5 μm in diameter (only 15 to 20% of its unstressed size). The membrane thickness is of the order of 70 to 100 Å, which gives a radius to thickness ratio of the order of 500. This means that the membrane is actually a thin shell and the thin shell theory is applicable to describe its behavior.

The red cell membrane is composed of 50 to 60% protein by dry weight, it is usually viewed as "double layer of long, relatively rigid molecules with their hydrophilic heads buried in the aqueous solutions on either side of the membrane and their hydrophobic tails isolated in the interior of the bilayer."[33] The remarkable deformability of the red blood cells and the capability of very large extension and a high bending stiffness is well-known. Aharon Katchalsky (Katzir) and his collaborators[34] were the first to obtain an analytical expression for the mechanical properties of the membrane. They assumed that the viscoelasticity of the red cell membrane can be represented by a Kelvin body with parallel viscous and elastic elements. This idea was later used by Rand,[47] who expanded the model, as shown in Figure 1 to describe the kinetic of membrane rupture. The expression for the tensile stress as a function of the mechanical parameters of Rand's model is given by:

$$\frac{1}{T} = \left[f \frac{1}{Y_2} + \frac{1}{Y_1} \left(1 - \exp\left(-\frac{Y_1}{\eta_1}t\right) \right) + \frac{1}{\eta_2} t \right] \tag{1}$$

where the parameters are described in Figure 1.

These models were later replaced by two different schools of thought. The one suggested by Chanham,[10] Chien et al.,[13] Skalak,[51] Brailsford and Bull,[1] and Zarda et al.[55] assumed a uniform shell with the shape of its geometry prescribed the minimum value of the membrane strain energy, associated with bending stiffness and shear rigidity. The other school of thought relates the red cell shape to its static equilibrium position as it is reached from the surface shear forces acting in the membrane, see Fung,[19] Fung and Tong,[20] and Evans.[16]

The analytical derivations of both these approaches are lengthy and tedious and the results are too complex to be included in the derivation of flow through the narrow vessels of the microcirculation. It is because of this reason that the analysis is omitted from this text, it is nevertheless an essential part of the mechanics of flow in the microcirculation.

C. Theories of Flow in the Microcirculation

The flow of blood in the smaller vessels of the microcirculation is highly complex and must be considered in a different approach than the flow of blood in the larger vessels. The blood can no longer be considered as a homogeneous suspension of cells in plasma. Instead the flow must be regarded as a two-phase system with plasma and red blood cells as the two phases. Although the white cells are much bigger than the red cells, they are not considered as the second phase because of the high ratio of red to white blood cells. Hence, the red cells are taken as the second phase ignoring the white cells and all other blood constituents. The number of cells passing through a specific capillary is not uniform, and at any instant there is a possibility of having one capillary with many cells, and another capillary in the same vascular bed with plasma only and no red blood cells. It is also possible that in a specific capillary the flow is halted for an undetermined period of time and then started again. The mechanism for this termination of flow is not known and is probably due to a local control mechanism and is not a result of the precapillary sphincter activity.

The Reynolds' number of flow through the capillary is of the order 10^{-2} to 10^{-3}. In this range of Reynolds' numbers, the inertia terms are much smaller than viscous stresses and pressure force and the flow can be considered as creeping flow with no inertia. Each capillary can be taken as an individual unit, since there is very little, if

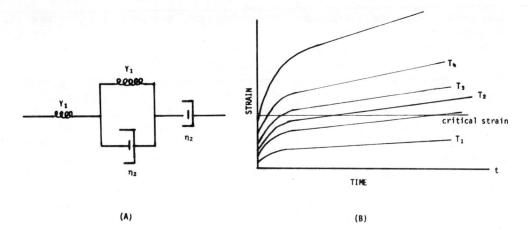

FIGURE 1.   (A) Mechanical viscoelastic model of the cell membrane. (B) The strain versus time behavior of the model for various stresses, using arbitrary viscous and elastic parameters. Y_1 and Y_2 are elastic parameters; n_1 and n_2 are viscous parameters.

any, interaction between adjacent capillaries. The blood vessels are taken with their immediate surrounding as a complete system of straight tube, relatively rigid with fluid exchange that is governed by the porosity of the endothelial layer and the diffusion across the basement membrane and the endothelial lining. The erythrocytes are moving within the capillary separated axially from one another by gaps filled with plasma. The size of these gaps varies both in space and with time. In the limit, when the axial gaps approach very small values, the line of red blood cells behave as a Rouleaux chain. The gaps separating successive cells are filled with plasma and are defined as a "bolus," a term suggested by Prothero and Burton.[45,46]

In the last two decades, the mechanism of flow and oxygen transport has attracted many scientists to try and describe the microcirculation as a system. Different analytical solutions were published in the literature for the flow of the red blood cell in the microcirculation. The major differences between these models are the assumptions about the geometry and mechanical properties of the erythrocyte and the nature of flow around them within the microvascular bed. The red blood cells were modeled as a rigid disk, see Goldsmith and Mason,[26] Fung,[21] Brenner and Bungay,[5] and many others; or as a liquid drop, see Guthier et al.,[23] and Kline;[35] or as a membrane with no bending moments, see Lin et al.,[41] and others. Different geometries were used for these models, most of them used for mathematical simplicity, like spherical geometry, see Bugliarello and Hsiao,[7] and Wang and Skalak;[53] or spheroidal both oblate and prolate, see Chen and Skalak;[12] or closer to reality geometries like elongated needles, see Lighthill;[39,40] or concave disks, see Bugliarello and Hsiao,[7] and Lin et al.[41] This different assumption changes not only the location at which boundary conditions are to be applied, but also the nature of the surface forces and the characteristics of the phenomenon. While rigid particles have only the no-slip conditions on their assumed surface geometry, the liquid drop involves surface tension as well as viscosity of the erythrocyte, which leads to deformation of the cell. The definition of a membrane implies no bending moments and only surface forces that act to deform the red cell when passing through the capillary.

During their passage through the narrow capillary tubes, the cells obtain a steady configuration and are moving with this deformed shape throughout the microcirculation. The solution to the flow equations can be that of Stokes flow around a chain of particles, or lubrication conditions between the red blood cells and the capillary wall.

It is also possible to use Poiseuille flow profiles with the red cell moving at a specific constant speed, other than the average blood velocities. In the radial gap between the erythrocyte and the vessel wall the conditions, for this case, are leading to a Couette-type solution.

In all the models the plasma is taken as viscous, imcompressible Newtonian fluid. The flow has a very low Reynolds' number so that creeping flow results, and the inertia terms are dropped from the equation. The fact that the flow is asymmetric allows for the introduction of Stokes stream function, which upon insertion of the appropriate boundary condition yields the Stokes flow over rigid particles in viscous fluid.

The Navier-Stokes equation for steady state without the inertial terms gives:

$$-\nabla \vec{P} + \mu \nabla^2 \vec{v} + \vec{f} = 0 \qquad (2)$$

where $\vec{f}$ is the vector describing forces per unit volume. The only possible forces are gravity and buoyancy. Although they are included in some of the published work, as for example Chen and Skalak,[12] they are very small and have no effect on the flow in the microcirculation, thus they can be omitted from the last equation. The velocity must obey the equation of continuity:

$$\nabla \vec{v} = 0 \qquad (3)$$

This set of equations is suitable for the use of a stream function Ψ, that satisfies the equation of continuity, and after insertion into the Navier-Stokes equation, yields

$$\nabla^4 \Psi = 0 \qquad (4)$$

The definition of Ψ depends upon the assumed geometry of the erythrocyte. In cylindrical coordinates, the relation between velocities and the stream function is given by:

$$v_z = -\frac{1}{r}\frac{\partial \Psi}{\partial r} \qquad v_r = \frac{1}{r}\frac{\partial \Psi}{\partial z} \qquad (5)$$

and Equation 4 is written as:

$$\left[\frac{\partial^2}{\partial z^2} - \frac{\partial^2}{\partial r^2} - \frac{1}{r}\frac{\partial}{\partial r}\right]^2 \Psi(r,z) = 0 \qquad (6)$$

while in spherical coordinates, the same equations are given by:

$$v_r = -\frac{1}{r^2 \sin\theta}\frac{\partial \Psi}{\partial \theta}$$

$$v_\theta = \frac{1}{r \sin\theta}\frac{\partial \Psi}{\partial r} \qquad (7)$$

while the more general case of ellipsoidal-shaped red cells, the equations are[12]

$$v_\lambda = \frac{1}{c^2 (\lambda^2 + \xi^2)^{1/2} (1 + \lambda^2)^{1/2}}\frac{\partial \Psi}{\partial \xi}$$

$$v_\xi = \frac{-1}{c^2 (\lambda^2 + \xi)^{1/2} (1 - \xi^2)^{1/2}}\frac{\partial \Psi}{\partial \lambda} \qquad (8)$$

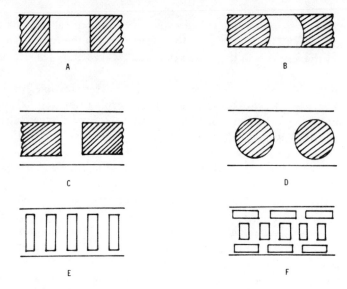

FIGURE 2.   Different assumed geometry of erythrocytes passing
through the microcirculation.(A and B, Bugliarello and Hsaio, 1970;
C, Bugliarello and Hsaio, 1970; Fung, 1973; D, Wang and Skalak,
1969; E, Lew and Fung, 1969; Huang, 1971; Lew, 1972; F, Lew,
1972.)

for oblate spheroidal coordinates, where (λ, ξ, ϕ) are the general orthogonal coordinates, and relate to tube cylindrical coordinates by:

$$R = C\lambda\xi \; ; \quad Z = C(\lambda^2 + 1)^{1/2} (1 - \xi^2)^{1/2} \; ; \quad \phi = \phi \qquad (9)$$

For prolate spheroidal coordinates the velocity components are given by:

$$v_\tau = \frac{1}{C^2 (\tau^2 - \xi^2)^{1/2} (\tau^2 - 1)^{1/2}} \frac{\partial \Psi}{\partial \xi}$$

$$v_\xi = \frac{1}{C^2 (\tau^2 - \xi^2)^{1/2} (1 - \xi^2)^{1/2}} \frac{\partial \Psi}{\partial \tau} \qquad (10)$$

With these relations the problem is now reduced to a solution of Equation 4 subject to appropriate boundary conditions. The boundary conditions are similar to all the geometries, except the different coordinate system for which they are written. The stream function must yield a given arbitrary particle velocity, U, on the surface of the erythrocyte, and a specific given rate of flow, Q. This rate of flow or discharge is computed on any cross section of the tube, and must give the same result, namely:

$$Q = -2\pi [\Psi]_{R = 1} \qquad (11)$$

where an adjustment is made to give $[\Psi]_{R=0} = 0$, so that the difference yields the last equation. In addition the flow near the wall is assumed to have no slip, thus giving:

$$v_z = 0 \;\; @ \;\; R = 1 \qquad (12)$$

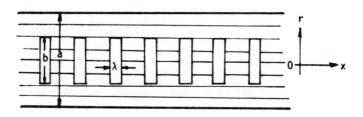

FIGURE 3.   Schematic diagram of approximated streamline in a simplified model of disc chain moving in a straight circular tube.

On the erythrocyte surface the boundary conditions must yield:

$$v_z = U \qquad v_R = 0 \tag{13}$$

In all the above-mentioned cases this is sufficient to solve Equation 4, and to use the other stream function relations to obtain the velocity components. The actual calculation is very lengthy and different for each coordinate system, and the reader is advised to use the reference mentioned earlier, and especially the detailed analysis described in Chen and Skalak.[12] From these solutions the pressure drop across the microcirculatory bed and the drag on each spheroid can be calculated.

Although the solution obtained in this tedious way is complex, and it is difficult to draw a clear-cut conclusion, it is possible to obtain one general assumption on the nature of flow. The major factor in the determination of pressure drop and drag is the ratio between the erythrocyte radial coordinate and the diameter of the tube. The exact particle shape and the number of particles per unit length, or unit volume, is only of a second order. If this assumption is used, it is reasonable to ignore the exact erythrocyte shape and to use an easier shape. And indeed, many investigators used this assumption, as shown in Figure 2.

As an example for the relation between pressure and flow in one of these simplified models, consider the solution suggested by Lew[37] for the case described in Figure 3. The flow is considered, as suggested before, with negligible viscosity (very small Re). The distance between two adjacent disks is much smaller than the radius of the tube, and the flow between the disks is assumed uniform and equal to the velocity of the disks. The radial velocity component in the plasma layer near the tube walls is taken as zero, although this is known to be incorrect. The only reason for this simplicity is the mathematical comfort. Thus, the following relations are used:

$$\left. \begin{array}{l} u = U \\ v = 0 \end{array} \right\} @ \ r{\le}b \qquad \left. \begin{array}{l} u = u(r) \\ v = 0 \end{array} \right\} @ \ r{>}b \tag{14}$$

This assumption leads to a pressure that depends only on the longitudinal coordinate and is the same as taking the pressure as uniform in any cross section. The Navier-Stokes equation for this case gives:

$$\frac{dP(x)}{dx} = \mu \, \frac{1}{r} \, \frac{\partial}{\partial r}\left(\frac{\partial u}{\partial r}\right) = \mu \, \frac{1}{r} \, \frac{du^2}{dr^2} \tag{15}$$

The solution for this equation is given by

$$u(r) = \frac{1}{\mu} \, \frac{dP}{dx}\left(\frac{r^2}{4} + A\ln r + B\right) \ r{>}b \tag{16}$$

where A and B are constants to be determined by the boundary conditions. The boundary conditions are u(r = a) = 0 and u(r = b) = U, but the particle velocity is not known. Writing the energy balance for a single disk gives:

$$\pi b^2 \left[P\left(-\frac{\lambda}{2}\right) - P\left(\frac{\lambda}{2}\right) \right] = 2\pi b\lambda\mu \frac{du}{dr} \ (r = b) \tag{17}$$

From the last two equations the velocity in the plasma layer and the particle velocity are obtained, as:

$$u(r) = \frac{1}{4\mu} \frac{dP}{dx} (a^2 - r^2) \quad r > b \tag{18}$$

$$U = -\frac{1}{4\mu} \frac{dP}{dx} (a^2 - b^2) \tag{19}$$

Equation 19 gives also the velocity of the plasmatic gap between two adjacent disks. There must, however, exist a relation between the number of particles and the plasma flow as the hematocrit must be the same at both ends of the capillary. So, the average velocity and disk volume must be calculated. The average velocity over a cross section is obtained by simple integration to yield:

$$<u> = -\frac{a^2}{8\mu} \frac{dP}{dx} \left(1 - \frac{b^4}{a^4} \right) \tag{20}$$

This shows that the average velocity is smaller than that obtained in Poiseuille flow, which indicates that the required pressure gradient is higher due to the existence of particles in the flow. The volume of N disks per unit length divided by the total volume gives the blood apparent hematocrit:

$$\Phi\text{app} = N \frac{\pi b^2 \lambda}{\pi a^2} = N\lambda \frac{b^2}{a^2} \tag{21a}$$

The effective hematocrit is obtained by dividing the volume of disks per unit length by the average velocity. Hence:

$$\Phi\text{eff} = \frac{UN\pi b^2 \lambda}{\frac{\pi}{2} U (a^2 + b^2)} = 2N\lambda \left(\frac{b^2}{a^2 + b^2} \right) \tag{21b}$$

and the ratio between the two hematocrits is given by:

$$\frac{\Phi_{\text{app}}}{\Phi_{\text{eff}}} = \frac{1}{2} \left(1 + \frac{b^2}{a^2} \right) \tag{22}$$

which indicates that the apparent hematocrit, if measured by photography, is much smaller than the real hematocrit. Thus, it is clear that not only the number of disks in each capillary at a unit time is not known *a priori,* but it cannot be calculated from volume ratio of erythrocytes and plasma.

The assumption of Couette-type flow in the plasma layer is arbitrary, and with the same basic assumptions other types of flows are also possible. Since the clearance is very small it is appropriate to apply lubrication theory. Lighthill[39,40] suggested the use

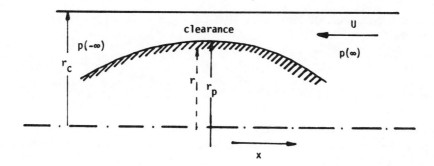

FIGURE 4.   Lighthill's model of tightly fitting pellets in fluid-filled elastic tube.

of hydrodynamic lubrication between the red blood cell and elastic tube walls. He assumed an elastic tube that can undergo radial deformation due to pressure differences and thus allowing particles with the same size as the tube diameter to pass through. After the particles are squeezed into the tube they move with a very small velocity. Lighthill's assumptions were

1.   The deformation of both wall and tube are linear with pressure. This assumption is essential to obtain an analytical solution, however it is far from true.
2.   The shape of the erythrocyte can be approximated by a parabolic profile.
3.   Each erythrocyte can be considered as a unit, thus regarding the whole problem as a single file. This is the major difference from the previous model of chain of particles since there is no interaction between cells.
4.   The capillary walls and the red blood cells are axisymmetric.
5.   There is no longitudinal tension which avoids the need for using the radius of curvature in the analysis.
6.   The clearance can be either positive or negative which permits all the possible displacements of the capillary wall and deformation of red blood cells.
7.   The pressure on both sides of the lubrication layer can be considered equal to the pressure in infinity.

With the geometry described in Figure 4 the undeformed state of the pellet can be described by:

$$r = r_0 - \frac{1}{2} kx^2 \tag{23}$$

where x is measured axially downstream from the point where the pellet cross section has its maximum radius r_0, and k is the curvature of the pellets at the points where the maximum radius is obtained. When pressure is applied the pellet is being deformed and the new geometry will depend linearly (as assumed) on the pressure difference. Hence:

$$r_p = r_0 - \frac{1}{2} kx^2 - \beta (P - P_0) \tag{24}$$

in the same way the radius of the capillary is given by:

$$r_c = r_0 + \alpha (P - P_0) \tag{25}$$

which gives a clearance, or lubricating film thickness h, between the pellet and the inner tube wall as:

$$h = (\alpha + \beta)(P - P_o) + \frac{1}{2} kx^2 \qquad (26)$$

where P_o is to be defined later, and the linearly parameters α and β are specific to the problem.

The assumption of hydrodynamic lubrication, namely the small and negligible inertia terms (relative to viscosity) and the existence of a boundary layer (the pressure is uniform in a cross section, and is therefore a function of x only) leads to the following governing equation:

$$\frac{dP}{dx} = \mu \frac{\partial^2 u}{\partial y^2} \qquad (27)$$

The y is a coordinate measured along the boundary layer. This equation must be solved subject to the following boundary conditions:

$$u(y = o) = 0; \quad u(y = h) = -U \qquad (28)$$

and the continuity equation:

$$\int_0^h u \, dy = -Q \qquad (29)$$

where Q represents the amount of back flow, and must be known in advance. The solution, for the Navier-Stokes equation subject to these boundary conditions, is given by:

$$\frac{u}{U} = 2\left[\frac{y}{h} - 3\left(\frac{y}{h}\right)^2\right] - \frac{6Q}{h}\left[\frac{y}{h} - \left(\frac{y}{h}\right)^2\right] \qquad (30)$$

and for the pressure gradient:

$$\frac{dP}{dx} = -\frac{6\mu U}{h} + \frac{6\mu Q}{h^2} \qquad (31)$$

This gives way to the calculation of shear stresses on the surface of the pellets and, hence, the drag acting on each particle as it is squeezed through the capillary.

$$\tau = -\mu\left(\frac{\partial u}{\partial y}\right)_{y=o} = -\frac{2\mu U}{h} + \frac{6\mu Q}{h^2} \qquad (32)$$

The total force is obtained by integration over the area of the pellet. This force must be balanced by pressure difference acting over the cross section. Lighthill assumed that h is small compared with r_o, and, hence, the equation for the balance of forces can be written as:

$$\P r_o^2 \left[P(-\infty) - P(+\infty)\right] = 2\P r_o \int_{-\infty}^{\infty} \tau \, dx = 2\P r_o \int_{-\infty}^{\infty} \left(-\frac{2\mu U}{h} + \frac{6\mu Q}{h^2}\right) dx \qquad (33)$$

Equations 32 and 33 introduce another limitation on the solution, since the solution must yield a positive shear stress and negative pressure gradients. This gives:

$$\frac{2Q}{U} < h < \frac{3Q}{U} \tag{34}$$

This limits the range of solutions, since for large (x), the clearance h must have a rather large value. However, this result is used by Lighthill to reduce the problem to a non-dimensional form by taking the lower value of h, namely 2Q/U as a typical film thickness. Thus reducing the problem to a nondimensional form by the following relations:

$$H = \frac{h}{2Q/U}$$

$$P = \frac{(\alpha + \beta)(P - P_o)}{2Q/U} \tag{35}$$

$$X = \left(\frac{k}{2Q/U}\right)^{1/2} x$$

The solutions can be written in nondimensional form as:

$$H = P + \frac{1}{2} X^2$$

$$\frac{dP}{dX} = L(H^{-3} - H^{-2}) \tag{36}$$

$$L = \frac{6\mu U(\alpha + \beta)}{(2Q/U)^{5/2} k^{1/2}}$$

And with introduction of a new parameter:

$$C = \frac{2Q}{Ur_o}$$

the ratio between the typical film thickness and the reference radius, the balance of forces is reduced to:

$$P(-\infty) - P(\infty) = LC \int_{-\infty}^{\infty} (H^{-2} - \frac{2}{3} H^{-1}) dX \tag{37}$$

Looking at Equation 36, one has, for the case where L is known, two different equations for H and P. So, if Q and U are known a solution can be obtained, however, the reference radius r_o is not determined at this stage. If the solution is known, together with the knowledge of the value of $P(\infty)$, it is possible to calculate $P(-\infty)$, and to use Equation 37 to find the value of C. The requirement for C to be positive and very small limits the band of possible solutions. Lighthill used perturbation techniques to solve for small and large values of L, and calculated numerically for values in the area between those expansions. Typical results are shown in Figures 5 and 6.

The importance of this model is in the definition of the possible ranges of the parameters α and β. Knowledge of these parameters can give a first approximation to more

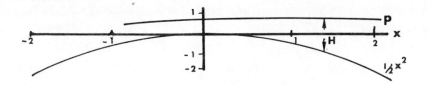

FIGURE 5.   The nondimensional pressure distribution P(x), clearance H and the function $(-\frac{1}{2}x^2)$, plotted as functions of the nondimensional axial coordinate X, for L = 1. (From Lighthill, M. J., *J. Fluid Mech.*, 34, 113, 1968. With permission.)

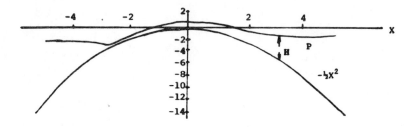

FIGURE 6.   The nondimensional pressure distribution P (x), clearance H and the function $(-\frac{1}{2}x^2)$, plotted as functions of the nondimensional axial coordinate X, for L = 8. (From Lighthill, M. J., *J. Fluid Mech.*, 34, 113, 1968. With permission.)

realistic assumptions on capillary wall and erythrocyte deformations as functions of pressure difference. However, some critical assumptions were made during his calculations that must be considered in more detail in further development of the model:

1.   The equation for pressure gradient in Equation 36 is assumed to be accurate enough so that the reversed curvature of both capillary wall and pellet can be neglected.
2.   The pellet edges can be taken as infinity both upstream and downstream.
3.   The shear stress in Equation 32 is sufficiently accurate to define the downstream pressure.

If Lighthill's results for small L are compared with the limit, which must approach Poiseuille's solution, it can be shown that this does not hold. It also gives very small value for the resistance and high value for clearance. However, it does not approach Poiseuille's solution. The possible explanation is that the second condition does not hold for this case. Fitz-Gerald[18] showed that in the case of small L, the error can be as high as 300%. He considered the same type of flow, writing the equation in cylindrical coordinates, and included the curvature of the capillary in his calculations.

Other models were suggested by many investigators, that differ mainly from the previous models by their assumed geometry. A very popular assumption used to be the parachute-shaped cells, this shape is reached due to deformation. In this model, Figure 7, the orientation of the parachute was usually assumed parallel to the capillary wall, an assumption that was used to convert the asymmetric problem to two-dimensional. Skalak and Branemark[52] suggested that this shape is the basic biconcave disk shape of the red blood cell. This shape can be justified by calculation of the elastic deformations, as discussed in the previous chapter.

It is clear, from observation of particle geometry, that the deformity of the red blood cell plays a major role in the determination of clearance. It is also a function of average blood velocity in the microcirculation, and in higher velocities the higher shear stress

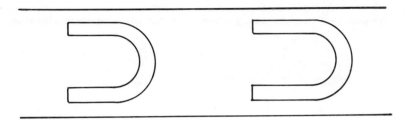

FIGURE 7. "Parachute" shape or biconcave disc shape of erythrocyte passing through the capillaries.

will cause a larger deformation and the particle will pass through the capillary with a larger clearance, as shown in Figure 8. The interaction of particle and the formation of larger aggregates is also of utmost importance and is discussed in more detail in the next chapter.

Another model, suggested by Howe and Sheaffer,[29] based upon observations of Heimberger,[28] Gibson et al.,[24] and Sapirstein,[49] considers the interstitial fluid in the tissue surrounding the capillary as an integral part of the capillary flow. The basic assumption in this model is that the capillary endothelium is not a barrier for the macromolecules, and hence for the plasma, and the real barrier lies outside the capillary at the edges of an annulus, called the Heimberger annulus. This barrier, the "true hematolymph barrier", is the actual boundary for the plasma flow, as shown in Figure 9. In this model the cells of radius $\bar{r}_1$ are moving inside a plasma filled annulus of radius $\bar{r}_3$, where the endothelium barrier equals $\bar{r}_2$. The momentum equation for slow viscous flow, with negligible inertia and asymmetric flow is:

$$\mu \frac{du^2}{dr^2} + \frac{\mu}{r} \frac{du}{dr} - \frac{dP}{dx} = 0 \qquad (38)$$

The balance of forces in the cylindrical train of cells, moving at uniform velocity $\bar{u}_c$ leads to the relation:

$$\frac{\bar{r}_1}{2} \frac{dP}{dx} = \left(\mu \frac{du}{dr}\right) \ r = \bar{r}_1 \qquad (39)$$

A solution to the momentum equation together with conditions of no-slip at the endothelial and true hematolymph barriers, and Equation 39, leads to the following velocity distribution:

$$u = -\frac{1}{4\mu} \frac{dP}{dx} (\bar{r}_2^2 - r^2) \quad \bar{r}_1 < r < \bar{r}_2 \qquad (40)$$

and

$$u_c = -\frac{1}{4\mu} \frac{dP}{dx} (\bar{r}_2^2 - \bar{r}_1^2) \qquad (41)$$

The total flow is obtained by integration of the velocity field across the cross section of the "enlarged tube" and the result is the following relations:

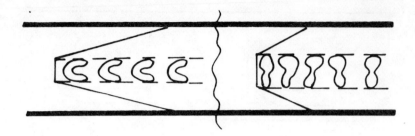

FIGURE 8.   Particle geometry and velocity distribution in blood flow in the micro-circulation. Low velocities on the left, and high velocities on the right.

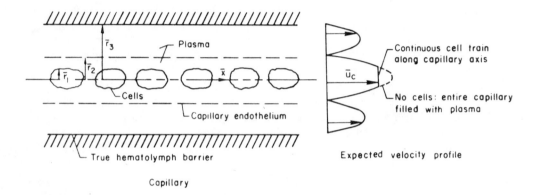

FIGURE 9.   A model of the hematolymph barrier for flow in a capillary and the expected velocity profile. (From Howe, J. T. and Sheaffer, Y. S., *NASA TN-D-3497,* 1966. With permission.)

$$Q_p = \pi \rho u_c \bar{r}_1^2 + \frac{\pi \rho}{8 \mu} \left(-\frac{dP}{dx} \right) (\bar{r}_2^2 - \bar{r}_1^2)^2$$

$$+ \frac{\pi \rho}{8 \mu} \left(-\frac{dP}{dx} \right) (\bar{r}_3^2 - \bar{r}_2^2). \tag{42}$$

$$\left\{ 2\bar{r}_3 - (\bar{r}_3^2 - \bar{r}_2^2) \left[1 + \frac{1}{\ln \bar{r}_3 / \bar{r}_2} \right] \right\}$$

for the flow of plasma, and if k is the fraction of cells train cylinder that is actually cells, the volume discharge of cells is:

$$Q_c = k \pi \rho u_c \bar{r}_1^2 \tag{43}$$

The hematocrit is thus given by:

$$h = Q_c \Big/ Q_p \tag{44}$$

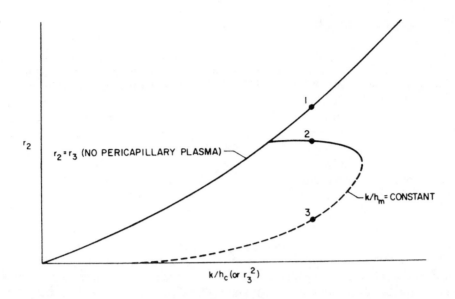

FIGURE 10. The region of possible solution to Equation 45. (From Howe, J. T. and Sheaffer, Y. S., *NASA TN-D-3497*, 1966. With permission.)

which results in the following relations:

$$\left[\left(\frac{k}{h_c}\right)^2 - \bar{r}_2^2 - (\bar{r}_2^2 - 1)\left(\frac{2k}{h} - 1\right)\right] \ln\left(\frac{\sqrt{k/h_c}}{\bar{r}_2}\right)$$

$$= \left(\frac{k}{h_c} - \bar{r}_2^2\right)^2 \qquad\qquad (45)$$

where h_c is defined as the dynamic hematocrit of the capillary, given by:

$$h_c = \frac{k}{\bar{r}_3^2} \qquad\qquad (46)$$

Howe and Sheaffer showed that there are three possible roots to the last equations. One, with $\bar{r}_2 = \bar{r}_3$, has no pericapillary flow, and the other two roots, $\bar{r}_2 < \bar{r}_3$, have pericapillary plasma. In the flow with pericapillary plasma, k/h remains constant, as shown in Figure 10. From this result they were able to show that spacing of erythrocyte is not always uniform, and that the cells are moving with a smaller velocity than the one obtained when no particles are present. It also explains how by enlarged plasmatic flow the capillary can adjust to accommodate variations in capillary flow. This model lacks the motion of fluid across the endothelial barrier, which results in different boundary conditions at this barrier, which is the topic of the next section.

D. Fluid Transport Across the Capillary Walls

The problem of transcapillary fluid exchange is much more complex and less is known about its mechanism than the problem of blood flow in capillaries. The exchange of fluids and other macromolecules across blood walls requires not only the knowledge of how the blood flows inside the capillaries, but also a knowledge of how the interstitial fluid moves through the tissue space, and what the driving forces and the local control in the flow are. The important species in transcapillary exchange are the proteins, however, they can be assumed to exist as a dilute soluble in plasma, thus comprising a single viscous and incompressible fluid.

It has been suggested by Starling in 1897 that the flow is determined by the balance between hydrostatic and protein osmotic pressures of the blood plasma. Starling's hypothesis is written as:

$$F.M = K(P_i - P_o + \pi_o - \pi_i) \tag{47}$$

where F.M is the mass rate of fluid mass movement across the capillary wall per unit area; P_i and P_o are the internal and external hydrostatic pressures, accordingly, and in the same way π_i and π_o are the internal and external protein osmotic pressures of the blood plasma. The linearity coefficient, K, is known as the permeability constant or the filtration constant and is measured by mass transferred per unit time, unit area and unit pressure. Despite its name, it is not a constant, but a function of the distance from the entrance of the capillary and in general, its value is different for the arterial or venous sides of the capillary. It is also not constant throughout the body and varies in different tissues, together with their protein's concentration. It should be noted that it has not been proven that the permeability coefficient for hydrostatic pressure equals that of osmotic pressure. The average normal range for the permeability constant is:

$$\text{(arterial) } (2 - 8)10^{-3} \text{ sec/cm} < K < (16 - 25)10^{-3} \text{ sec/cm (venous)}$$

In general this equation is nonlinear since, for example, the pressure outside the capillary, P_o, is determined by the interstitial fluid volume which itself depends upon the capillary pressure, the osmotic pressure, the permeability of the capillary and the lymph flow. So the parameters are interconnected in a complicated way that, because of lack of further knowledge, was left out of most of the published works. To analyze mathematically the fluid exchange across the capillary flow, few additional assumptions are necessary. The capillary joining the arteriole with the venule is taken as a straight rigid tube of circular cross section and finite length L. Apelblat et al.[3] considered the flow in a conical capillary taking into consideration the known fact that the area available for fluid exchange is larger on the venous side. However, in their analysis they did not consider the influence of the surrounding tissue space. The tissue space is considered as a space of infinite extent. The fluid flow through the capillary wall flows according to Starling's hypothesis, however, the rate of flow through the wall is much smaller than the rate of flow through the tube. The hydrostatic interstitial fluid pressure is assumed constant. Intaglietta[32] showed that that is not true and that the filtration coefficient increases significantly from the arterial to venous ends of the capillary. Wiederhielm[54] obtained the same results. The blood is a homogenous, incompressible, and Newtonian fluid and the flow is laminar and axisymmetric, with inertia terms much smaller than viscous terms, and no body forces. The entrance and outlet conditions are ignored and the pressure in the venule is determined by the flow properties and the entrance arterial pressure. The boundary conditions at the wall are taken to be the no-slip conditions, and the thickness of the capillary wall is assumed to be very small, so that boundary conditions for the capillary and for the surrounding tissue can

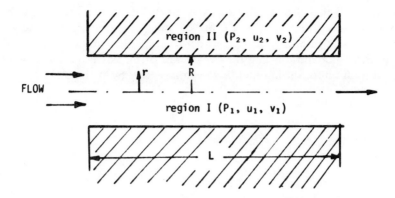

FIGURE 11.   The geometry of a single capillary (Region I) and the surrounding tissues (Region II).

be taken to be in the same location. The geometry of the problem is shown in Figure 11.

In both regions the equations of continuity and momentum must be satisfied, hence,

continuity

$$\frac{1}{r}\frac{\partial}{\partial r}(rv_i) + \frac{\partial u_i}{\partial z} = 0 \tag{48}$$

momentum

$$\frac{\partial P_i}{\partial r} = \mu\left(\frac{\partial^2 v_i}{\partial r^2} + \frac{1}{r}\frac{\partial v_i}{\partial r} - \frac{v_i}{r} + \frac{\partial^2 v_i}{\partial z^2}\right)$$

$$\frac{\partial P_i}{\partial z} = \mu\left(\frac{\partial^2 u_i}{\partial r^2} + \frac{1}{r}\frac{\partial u_i}{\partial r} + \frac{\partial^2 u_i}{\partial z^2}\right) \tag{49}$$

where v is the radial velocity component and u is the longitudinal velocity component, written in cylindrical coordinate system, and $i = 1$ is for Region I and $i = 2$ for Region II.

The boundary conditions are

$$\frac{\partial u_1}{\partial r} = 0 ; \qquad v_1 = 0 \quad \text{at} \quad r = 0$$

$$u_1 = 0 ; \quad u_2 = 0 ; \quad v_1 = v_2 = k(P_1 - P_2 - \alpha) \quad \text{at} \quad r = R$$

$$u_2 = 0 ; \qquad \overline{P}_1 = P_a \quad \text{at} \quad z = 0 \tag{50}$$

$$u_2 = 0 ; \qquad \overline{P}_1 = P_v \quad \text{at} \quad z = L$$

where $\alpha = \pi_2 - \pi_2$ is the driving osmotic pressure difference, P_a and P_v are the arterial and venous blood pressures, and $\overline{P}_1$ denotes an average over the cross section of the pressure.

It was assumed that the radial velocity is much smaller than the longitudinal one, so it can be assumed that u, v, and P are of order 1, ϵ and 1, respectively, and that the derivatives with respect to z are of order ϵ compared with derivatives with respect to r. With these assumptions and the expansions of the equations and boundary conditions, the solution for the internal flow region is given by Dinnar:[15]

$$u = -\frac{1}{4\mu}\frac{dP_{11}}{dz}(R^2 - r^2) + \frac{1}{32\mu}\frac{d^3P_{11}}{dz^3}(R^4 - r^4)$$

$$\cdot\,\frac{\alpha(z)}{4}(R^2 - r^2) + \sigma(\epsilon)$$

$$v = \frac{1}{16\mu}\frac{d^2P_{11}}{dz^2}(2rR^2 - r^3) - \frac{1}{320\mu}\frac{d^4P_{11}}{dz^4}(5rR^4 - 2r^5) \qquad (51)$$

$$-\frac{1}{16}\frac{d\alpha}{dz}(2rR^2 - r^3)$$

$$P = P_{11} + \sigma(\epsilon)$$

where P_{11} and $\alpha(z)$ are functions that are to be determined by matching this solution and the solution in Region II. The pressure inside the capillary is to the first order, a function of z only; it is reasonable to assume that the hydrostatic pressure in the tissue P_{11} can be taken as a function of z only. Hence, the governing equations for Region II are

$$\frac{\partial^2 v_2}{\partial r^2} + \frac{1}{r}\frac{\partial v_2}{\partial r} - \frac{v_2}{r_2} + \frac{\partial^2 v_2}{\partial z^2} = 0$$

$$\frac{dP_2}{dz} = \mu\left(\frac{\partial^2 u_2}{\partial r_2} + \frac{1}{r}\frac{\partial u_2}{\partial r} + \frac{\partial^2 u_2}{\partial z^2}\right) \qquad (52)$$

$$\frac{1}{r}\frac{\partial}{\partial r}(rv_2) + \frac{\partial u_2}{\partial z} = 0$$

By using a separation of variables

$$v_2 = \rho(r)\,Z(z) \qquad (53)$$

the general solution to Equation 51 is given by:

$$u_2 = \sum_{n=1}^{\infty}\left[a_n J_0(\lambda_n r) + b_n Y_0(\lambda_n r)\right]\left[c_n e^{\lambda_n z} - d_n e^{-\lambda_n z}\right]$$

$$+ g_1(Z^2 + 2AZ) + h(r)$$

$$v_2 = \sum_{n=1}^{\infty}\left[a_n J_1(\lambda_n r) + b_n Y_1(\lambda_n r)\right]\left[c_n e^{\lambda_n z} + d_n e^{-\lambda_n z}\right] \qquad (54)$$

$$+\left(g_1 r + \frac{g_2}{r}\right)(Z + A)$$

where J_0, Y_0, J_1, Y_1 are Bessel function of the first and second kind, λ_n are the eigenvalues which will be determined by the matched boundary conditions, g_1, g_2, and A are constant, and h(r) is a compensation function that will yield $P_2 = P_2(Z)$.

By introduction of the boundary conditions and the matched boundary conditions the general solution can be found. If the equations are nondimensionalized by the introduction of the longitudinal Poiseuille flow, given by:

$$u_p = \frac{(P_a - P_v)R^2}{4\mu L} \tag{55}$$

and introduction of:

$$\Phi = \frac{P}{P_a}; \quad \zeta = \frac{Z}{L}; \quad \rho = \frac{r}{R}; \quad h = \frac{P_{20} + \alpha}{P_a}$$

$$u^\star = \frac{u}{u_p}; \quad v^\star = {v}/{u_p}; \quad \delta = \left[\frac{16k\mu L^2}{R^3}\right]^{1/2} \tag{56}$$

the general solution is given by:

$$u_1^\star = -\delta\left[Ee^{\delta\zeta} - Fe^{-\delta\zeta}\right]\left\{(1 - \rho^2) - \frac{\delta^2\epsilon^2}{8}(1 - \rho^4)\right\}$$

$$v_1^\star = \frac{\delta^2\epsilon}{4}\left[Ee^{\zeta\delta} + Fe^{-\delta\zeta}\right]\rho\left\{(2 - \rho^2) - \frac{\delta^2\epsilon^3}{12}(3 - \rho^4)\right\}$$

$$\phi_1 = h + \left[Ee^{\delta\zeta} + Fe^{-\delta\zeta}\right]\left\{1 - \frac{\delta^2\epsilon^3}{4}(1 + \rho^2)\right\}\left(\frac{P_a - P_v}{P_a}\right) \tag{57}$$

$$u_2^\star = -\frac{1}{4}\delta^2\epsilon\frac{Y_0(\delta\epsilon)J_0(\delta\epsilon\rho) - Y_0(\delta\epsilon\rho)J_0(\delta\epsilon)}{Y_0(\delta\epsilon)J_1(\delta\epsilon) - Y_1(\delta\epsilon)J_0(\delta\epsilon)}\left[Ee^{\delta\zeta} - Fe^{-\delta\zeta}\right]$$

$$v^\star = \frac{1}{4}\delta^2\epsilon\frac{Y_0(\delta\epsilon)J_1(\delta\epsilon\rho) - Y_1(\delta\epsilon\rho)J_0(\delta\epsilon)}{Y_0(\delta\epsilon)J_1(\delta\epsilon) - Y_1(\delta\epsilon)J_0(\delta\epsilon)}\left[Ee^{\delta\zeta} + Fe^{-\delta\zeta}\right]$$

$$\phi_2 = h - \alpha$$

and the constants E and F are given by:

$$E = \frac{P_a}{P_a - P_v}\frac{(e^{-\delta} - (P_v/P_a)) - h(e^{-\delta} - 1)}{e^\delta - e^{-\delta}}$$

$$\tag{58}$$

$$F = \frac{P_a}{P_a - P_v}\frac{(e^{-\delta} - (P_v/P_a)) - h(e^{-\delta} - 1)}{e^\delta - e^{-\delta}}$$

In the limit as $\delta \to 0$, which means $k \to 0$, there is no fluid exchange across the wall, this solution is then reduced to the simple Poiseuille flow.

The longitudinal and radial velocity distribution is described in Figures 12 and 13. It can be seen immediately that at a specific point ζ_1 along the capillary there is a zero radial flow. From the entry to this point there is a net outflow from the capillary into the surrounding tissues, and from this point on there is a drainage of fluid from the surrounding tissue into the capillary. It is thus possible, by calculation of ζ_1, to define

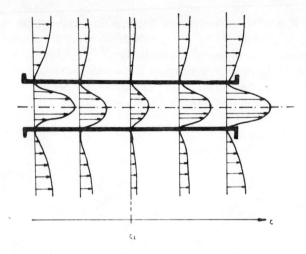

FIGURE 12.   Longitudinal velocity distribution (with minimum occurring at $\zeta = \zeta_0$). (From Dinnar, U., *Israel J. Tech.,* 10, 315, 1972. With permission.)

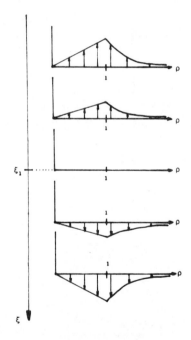

FIGURE 13.   Radial velocity distribution (with zero radial velocity at $\zeta - \zeta_1$). (From Dinnar, U., *Israel J. Tech.,* 10, 315, 1972. With permission.)

the transition from arterial behavior of the capillary and venous behavior. The point of transition is given by:

$$\zeta_1 = \frac{P_a - (P_{20} + \alpha)}{P_a - P_v} \qquad (59)$$

which is predetermined by the arterial, venous, and osmotic pressure. For equilibrium conditions, namely equal rates of inflow and outflow from the capillary ζ_1 has to equal

½, which can determine $P_{20} + \alpha$ for normal conditions. This value agrees well with experimental results obtained by many researchers.

Another interesting result of this model is the fact that it is impossible by an increase of P_{20}, the interstitial fluid pressure, to occlude the capillary (make $u_1 = 0$ at $\zeta = 0$). This shows that the local control of cessation of flow in a specific capillary can be only in the arterial and venous pressure and not in the interstitial fluid pressure or the osmotic pressure difference. This can, however, change the rate of flow, but not to stop the flow completely.

Similar models were suggested by Oka and Murata,[44] Apelblat et al.,[3] Murata,[42] Salathe and An,[48] and others.

E. Transcapillary Exchange by Diffusion

In the previous analysis the blood was considered as an homogenous medium. This simplifies the process and its mathematical description. However, the red blood cell flowing inside the capillary is a carrier of many small macromolecules, and the interesting phenomenon is the transfer of these molecules to the surrounding tissue. This is being done in two steps. In the first step the substrate is being transported into the surrounding tissue by both diffusion and convection. However, in general it is assumed that the diffusion across the capillary membrane is the most significant contributor to the transport mechanism. This transfer is only bound by the change in concentration of a particular specie and the restriction of the capillary wall pores to transfer of molecules with dimensions that are too large. The convection by the mechanism of Starling's hypothesis results in a flux which is of a smaller order and is usually considered as a correction to the diffusion transfer.

The first theoretical investigation of the oxygen transfer by diffusion has been made by Krogh,[36] by considering an infinitely long cylindrical tube surrounded by concentric cylinder of homogeneous tissue. This geometry is known as the Krogh cylinder and further assumed constant rate of oxygen consumption at the tissue and constant diffusion coefficients in the tissue. With this model it is possible to work with flow properties inside the capillary with concentration of oxygen or any other insoluble molecule. Inside the tissue the substrate movements by diffusion and by convection can be related to the concentration of substrate and written in cylindrical coordinates (r, θ, z) as:

$$\frac{\partial c}{\partial t} = \frac{1}{r}\frac{\partial}{\partial r}\left(rD_r\frac{\partial c}{\partial r}\right) + \frac{\partial}{\partial z}\left(D_z\frac{\partial c}{\partial z}\right) + \frac{1}{r^2}\frac{\partial}{\partial \theta}\left(D_\theta\frac{\partial c}{\partial \theta}\right) - Q(c) \tag{60}$$

where D_r, D_θ and D_z are the diffusion coefficients in the r, θ, and z direction, respectively; c is the concentration of the substrate and $Q(c)$ is a function of substrate concentration and describes the time rate for production or consumption of the substrate per unit volume.

Although this equation is basically for insoluble molecules, they are often used for all kinds of molecules, and in many cases for the oxygen concentration, even inside the capillary, thus ignoring the biochemical processes of oxygen transfer from hemoglobin to plasma and the reaction that is taking place inside the tissues. The function of fluid consumption, $Q(c)$, can be expanded to include the plasma flow inside the capillary. When this equation is used for the interior of the capillary the equations for velocity distribution must be included, as they are the major contributor to substrate convection.

For lack of knowledge it is logical to assume that the diffusion coefficients are the same in all directions, which is equivalent to the assumption of homogeneous diffusion. Under this assumption there is a justification to assume cylindrical symmetry. Hence, the partial differential equation for soluble or insoluble material concentration in the tissue domain is reduced to:

$$\frac{\partial c}{\partial t} = D\left(\frac{1}{r}\frac{\partial c}{\partial r} + \frac{\partial^2 c}{\partial r^2} + \frac{\partial^2 c}{\partial z^2}\right) - Q(c) \tag{61}$$

The relation for the substrate concentration function is usually taken to follow the Michaelis Menten enzyme substrate kinetics, for example Gonzalez-Fernandez and Atta:[27]

$$Q(c) = \frac{K_1 c}{K_2 + C} \tag{62}$$

where K_1 and K_2 are constants and are always positive.

For fully developed laminar flow in the capillary it is usually assumed that the velocity profile is parabolic, which is known to be very far from reality. It is, however, assumed for mathematical simplicity. Under these assumptions the equation for the concentration of substrate inside the capillary is given by the partial differential equation:

$$\frac{\partial c}{\partial t} = D\left(\frac{1}{r}\frac{\partial c}{\partial r} + \frac{\partial^2 c}{\partial r^2} + \frac{\partial^2 c}{\partial z^2}\right) - u_0\left(1 - \frac{r^2}{R^2}\right)\frac{\partial c}{\partial x} \tag{63}$$

where the function $Q(c)$ is replaced by a convection term.

Another possibility to include convection in the equation is to replace the partial derivative with respect to time, $\partial c/\partial t$, by the convected derivative Dc/Dt.

In writing the boundary conditions for these equations the inlet conditions are assumed uniform with symmetry at both the arterial and venous sides, thus leading to the following boundary conditions:

$$c(t, o, r) = c_a \quad t \geq 0$$
$$c(t, L, r) = c_r \quad t \geq 0 \tag{64}$$

The second boundary condition is replaced, in most published works, by a condition in infinity, namely:

$$c(t, \infty, r) = 0 \quad t \geq 0 \tag{65}$$

Krogh's original boundary conditions were taken as:

$$\frac{\partial c}{\partial z} = 0, \quad \text{for } 0 \leq r \leq R \quad z = 0 \quad \text{and} \quad z = L \tag{66}$$

The initial conditions are taken as:

$$c(0, z, r) = 0 \quad z \geq 0 \tag{67}$$

and balance equation at the boundary common to the capillary and tissue is given by:

$$\pi R^2 \bar{u} c = 2\pi RD \left(\frac{\partial c}{\partial r}\right)_{r=R} \tag{68}$$

where $\bar{u}$ is the cross-sectional average velocity. Gonzalez-Fernandez and Atta[27] replaced the concentration on the left-hand side by a function that includes the dissociation of oxygen and the cross-sectional average blood concentration of dissolved oxygen.

Krogh's original solution to this problem is based on the assumption of steady state conditions with neglected axial diffusion and metabolic rate which is independent of the concentration conditions. Under these assumptions, and uniform oxygen content at the axial and radial direction, the equation of substrate concentration is reduced to:

$$\frac{1}{r}\left(\frac{d}{dr}\left(r\frac{dc}{dr}\right)\right) = \frac{g_0}{D} \tag{69}$$

The solution requires only two boundary conditions, at the capillary boundary R, and at the tissue boundary R_T, namely:

$$c = c_0 \quad \text{at} \quad r = R$$

$$\frac{\partial c}{\partial r} = 0 \quad \text{at} \quad r = R_T \tag{70}$$

$$c = c + \frac{g_0}{D}\left(\frac{r^2 - R^2}{4} - \frac{R_T^2}{2}\ln\frac{r}{R}\right) \tag{71}$$

This solution, known as the Krogh single capillary solution, was later expanded to include all the other conditions mentioned above. Davis and Parkinson[14] used the same basic assumption, but changed the metabolic rate term to include the convection. Thus inside the capillary they obtained the dimensionless equation:

$$\frac{1}{\rho}\frac{\partial c}{\partial \rho} + \frac{\partial^2 c}{\partial \rho^2} = \frac{u(\rho)}{2}\frac{\partial c}{\partial \zeta} \tag{72}$$

where the dimensionless variables are defined as:

$$\rho = \frac{r}{R}; \quad \zeta = \frac{z}{RP_e}; \quad u(\rho) = \frac{u(r)}{u_m}; \quad c = \frac{c(r, z) - cd}{c_{in} - c_d} \tag{73}$$

where c_{in} is inlet concentration, C_d the external concentration, u_m is the mean velocity and P_e is Peclet number that describes the ratio between mean axial flow and diffusion, and is given by:

$$P_e = \frac{u_m R}{D} \tag{74}$$

The previous boundary conditions, written in dimensionless form are

$$c(\rho) = 1 \qquad 0 \leqslant \rho \leqslant 1 \qquad \zeta = 0$$

$$c(\rho) = 0 \qquad 0 \leqslant \rho \leqslant 1 \qquad \zeta \to \infty \tag{75}$$

$$\frac{\partial c(\rho)}{\partial \rho} = -Sh_w c(\rho) \qquad \rho = 1$$

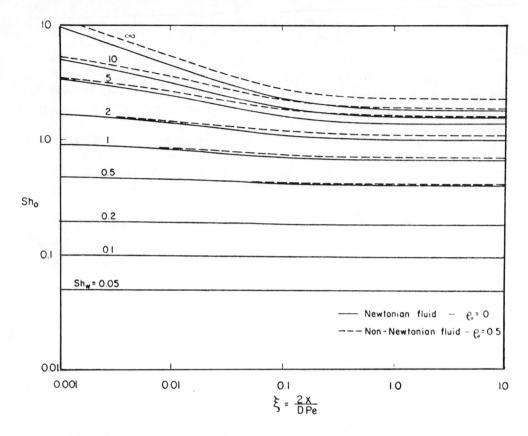

Sh$_o$

FIGURE 14.   Overall Sherwood number for Newtonian and Casson fluids under various conditions of wall resistance. (From Davis, M. R. and Parkinson, G. V., *Appl. Sci. Res.,* 22, 20, 1970. With permission.)

where sh$_w$ is the wall Sherwood number, relating the wall permeability P, and diffusion, and is given by:

$$Sh_w = \frac{PR}{D} \qquad\qquad (76)$$

The solution to the equation and the boundary conditions are obtained by separation of variables. This reduces the problem to a well-known heat transfer problem known as the Graetz problem. Davis and Parkinson used this method to compare between Newtonian and Casson's fluids and showed that the overall Sherwood number, given by Sh$_o$ = hR/D, where h is the overall mass transfer coefficient, varies only slightly in the non-Newtonian case, as shown in Figure 14.

There are many numerical solutions to this problem. A full description of them would be too lengthy, thus only two such examples are referenced for further reading, Ananthakrishnan et al.,[2] Gill and Ananthakrishnan,[25] and Gonzalez-Fernandez and Atta.[27]

A treatment of the same problem using electrical analog is given by Aberg and Hagglund.[1]

REFERENCES

1. Aberg, B. and Hagglund, J. V., A convection-diffusion model of capillary permeability with reference to single injection experiments, *Uppsala J. Med. Sci.*, 79, 7, 1974.
2. Ananthakrishnan, V., Gill, W. N., and Barduhn, A. J., Laminar dispersion in capillaries. Mathematical analysis, *AIChE J.*, 1063, 1965.
3. Apelblat, A., Katzir-Katchalsky, A., and Silberberg, A., A mathematical analysis of capillary-tissue fluid exchange, *Biorheology*, 11, 1, 1974.
4. Azuma, T. and Oka, S., Mechanical equilibrium of blood vessel wall, *Am. J. Physiol.*, 221, 1310, 1971.
5. Brenner, H. and Bungay, P. M., Rigid-particle and liquid-drop models of red cell motion in capillary tubes, *Fed. Proc.*, 30, 1565, 1971.
6. Brailsford, J. D. and Bull, B. S., The red cell-a macro model simulating the hypotonic-sphere isotonic-disc transformation, *J. Theor. Biol.*, 39, 325, 1973.
7. Bugliarello, G. and Hsiao, G. C., A mathematical model of the flow in the axial plasmatic gaps of the smaller vessels, *Biorheology*, 7, 5, 1970.
8. Burton, A. C., On the physical equilibrium of small blood vessels, *Am. J. Physiol.*, 164, 319, 1951.
9. Burton, A. C. and Yamada, S., Relation between blood pressure and flow in the human forearm, *J. Appl. Physiol.*, 4, 329, 1951.
10. Chanham, P. B., The minimum energy of bending as a possible explanation of the biconcave shape of the human red blood cells, *J. Theor. Biol.*, 26, 61, 1970.
11. Charm, S. E. and Kurland, G. S., *Blood Flow and Microcirculation*, John Wiley & Sons, New York, 1974.
12. Chen, T. C. and Skalak, R., Stokes flow in a cylindrical tube containing a line of spheroidal particles, *Appl. Sci. Res.*, 22, 403, 1970.
13. Chien, S., Luse, S. A., and Bryand, C. A., Hemolysis during filtration through micropores: a scanning electron microscopic and hemorhealogic correlation, *Microvasc. Res.*, 3, 183, 1971.
14. Davis, M. R. and Parkinson, G. V., Mass transfer from small capillaries with wall resistance in the laminar flow regime, *Appl. Sci. Res.*, 22, 20, 1970.
15. Dinnar, U., Simplified model for the exchange of fluid across the walls of a permeable capillary in blood circulation, *Israel J. Technol.*, 10, 315, 1972.
16. Evans, E. A., New membrane concept applied to the analysis of fluid shear- and micropipette-deformed red blood cells, *Biophys. J.*, 13, 941, 1973.
17. Evans, E. A., Waugh, R., and Melnik, L., Elastic area compressibility modulus of red cell membrane, *Biophys. J.*, 16, 585, 1976.
18. Fitz-Gerald, J. M., Mechanics of red-cell motion through very narrow capillaries, *Proc. R. Soc. London Ser. B*, 174, 193, 1969.
19. Fung, Y. C., Theoretical consideration of the elasticity of red cells and small blood vessels, *Fed. Proc.*, 25, 1761, 1966.
20. Fung, Y. C. and Tong, P., Theory of sphering of red blood cells, *Biophys. J.*, 8, 175, 1968.
21. Fung, Y. C., Blood flow in the capillary bed, *J. Biomech.*, 2, 353, 1969.
22. Fung, Y. C., Stochastic flow in capillary blood vessels, *Microvasc. Res.*, 5, 34, 1973.
23. Gauthrer, F. J., Goldsmith, H. L., and Mason, S. G., Flow of suspensions through tubes-X: liquid drops as models of erythrocytes, *Biorheology*, 9, 205, 1972.
24. Gibson, W. P., Bosley, P., and Griffiths, R., Photomicrographic studies on the nail bed capillary networks in human control subjects, *J. Nerv. Ment. Dis.*, 123, 219, 1956.
25. Gill, W. N. and Ananthakrishnan, V., Laminar dispersion in capillaries. Effect of inlet boundary conditions and Turner type of system capacitance, *AIChE J.*, 906, 1966.
26. Goldsmith, H. L. and Mason, S. G., The microrheology of dispersions, in *Rheology*, Eirich, F. R., Ed., Vol. 4, Academic Press, New York, 1967, 83.
27. Gonzalez-Fernandez, J. M. and Atta, S. E., Transport and consumption of oxygen in capillary-tissue structures, *Math. Biosci.*, 2, 225, 1968.
28. Heimberger, H., Kontraktik Function and Anatomischer bas a der Menschlichen Kapillaren, *Z. Zellforsch. Mikrosk. Anat.*, 4, 713, 1926.
29. Howe, J. T. and Sheaffer, Y. S., On the dynamics of capillaries and the existence of plasma flow in the pericapillary lymph space, *NASA Tech. Note*, TN-D-3497, 1966.
30. Huang, H. K., Theoretical analysis of flow patterns in single-file capillaries, *J. Biomech.*, 4, 103, 1971.
31. Hung, T. K., Weissman, M. H., and Bugliarello, G., A numerical model for two-dimensional oscillatory flow and oxygen transfer in the axial plasmatic gaps of capillaries, in *Theoretical and Clinical Hemorheology*, Hartret, H. H. and Copley, A., Eds., Springer-Verlag, Basel, 1971, 60.

32. Intaglietta, M., Evidence for a gradient of permeability in frog mesenteric capillaries, *Bibl. Anat.*, 9, 465, 1967.

33. Jenkins, J. T., Static equilibrium configuration of a model red blood cell, *J. Math. Biol.*, 4, 149, 1977.

34. Katchalsky, A., Kedem, O., Klibansky, C., and DeVries, A., Rheological considerations of the hae-molyzing red blood cell, in *Flow Properties of Blood and Other Biological Systems*, Copley, A. L. and Stainsby, G., Eds., Pergamon Press, Elmsford, N.Y., 1960, 155.

35. Kline, K. A., On a liquid drop model of blood rheology, *Biorheology*, 9, 287, 1972.

36. Krogh, A., The number and distribution of capillaries in muscles with calculation of the oxygen pressure head necessary for supplying, *J. Physiol. (London)*, 52, 409, 1919.

37. Lew, H. S., An arithmetical approach to the mechanics of blood flow in small caliber blood vessels, *J. Biomech.*, 5, 49, 1972.

38. Lew, H. S. and Fung, Y. C., The motion of the plasma between the red cells in the Bolus flow, *Biorheology*, 6, 109, 1969.

39. Lighthill, M. J., Pressure-forcing of lightly fitting pellets along fluid-filled elastic tubes, *J. Fluid Mech.*, 34, 113, 1968.

40. Lighthill, M. J., Motion in narrow capillaries from the standpoint of lubrication theory, in *Circula-tory and Respiratory Mass Transport*, Wolstenholme, G. E. W. and Knight, J., Eds., Little, Brown, Boston, 1969, 85.

41. Lin, K. L., Lupez, L., and Hellums, J. D., Blood flow in capillaries, *Microvasc. Res.*, 5, 7, 1973.

42. Murata, T., A theoretical analysis of material transport across a capillary wall, *Jpn. J. Appl. Phys.*, 14, 549, 1975.

43. Nichol, J., Girling, F., Jerrand, W., Claxton, E. B., and Burton, A. C., Fundamental instability of small blood vessels and critical closing pressure in vascular beds, *Am. J. Physiol.*, 164, 330, 1951.

44. Oka, S. and Murata, T., A theoretical study of the flow of blood in capillary with permeable wall, *Jpn. J. Appl. Phys.*, 9, 345, 1970.

45. Prothero, J. W. and Burton, A. C., The physics of blood flow in capillaries. I. The nature of the motion, *Biophys. J.*, 1, 565, 1961.

46. Prothero, J. W. and Burton, A. C., Physics of blood flow in capillaries. II. The capillary resistance to flow, *Biophys. J.*, 2, 199, 1962.

47. Rand, R. P., Mechanical properties of the red cell membrane. II. Viscoelastic breakdown of the membrane, *Biophys. J.*, 4, 303, 1964.

48. Salathe, E. P. and An, K. N., A mathematical analysis of fluid movement across capillary walls, *Microvasc. Res.*, 11, 1, 1976.

49. Sapirstein, L., Macromolecular exchanges in capillaries, in *The Microcirculation*, University of Illi-nois Press, Urbana, 1958, 47.

50. Skalak, R., Mechanics of the microcirculation, in *Biomechanics, Its Foundation and Objectives*, Fung, Y. C., Ed., Prentice-Hall, Englewood Cliffs, N.J., 1972, 457.

51. Skalak, R., Modeling mechanical behavior of red blood cells, *Biorheology*, 10, 229, 1973.

52. Skalak, R. and Branemark, P. I., Deformation of red blood cells in capillaries, *Science*, 164, 717, 1969.

53. Wang, H. and Skalak, R., Viscous flow in a cylindrical tube containing a line of spherical particles, *J. Fluid Mech.*, 38, 75, 1969.

54. Wiederhielm, C. A., Analysis of small vessel function, in *Physical Bases of Circulatory Transport: Regulation and Exchange*, Reeve, E. B. and Guyton, A. C., Eds., W. B. Saunders, Philadelphia, 1967, 313.

55. Zarda, P. R., Chein, S., and Skalak, R., Elastic deformation of red blood cells, *J. Biomech.*, 10, 211, 1977.

Chapter 10

FLUID MECHANICS OF THROMBUS FORMATION

A. Introduction

Thrombus, a Greek word meaning lump or clot, is used to describe a mass of cells and tissues that forms within the vascular system. Although this mass can sometimes contain fragments of tumors or other kinds of tissues, it mainly refers to a mass of blood constituents that are abstracted from the blood passing the thrombi. The process of formation of thrombus, known as thrombosis, is an essential mechanism in the process of hemostasis. The hemostasis process is an intravascular-triggered mechanism to protect the vascular system from leaks and thus protect its integrity. The process involves different phenomena that not only overlap one another but interact with one another in a very complex manner. These phenomena are adhesion of platelets to a region of intravascular damage (wound, destruction of endothelial layer), the formation of platelets plugs, the absorption of fibrin into the platelet plug, and the removal of deposited material by different mechanisms. Although the initial steps of thrombosis are similar in various parts of the circulation, the mechanisms are different in the formation of venous thrombi or arterial thrombi. The formation of venous thrombi is closer to that of blood coagulation and consists mainly of trapped red blood cells and fibrin. The arterial thrombi on the other hand has a different structure and is composed of a first layer of platelet aggregate with layers of fibrin and trapped blood cells are subsequently deposited. Paterson[22] pointed out that venous thrombi, similar in structure to that of the arterial thrombi, can be found in the pockets of vein valves, where the flow conditions might be very sluggish, especially in patients who undergo surgery or are immobile in bed for long periods. The formation period of thrombi is only a few seconds which makes it very hard to experimentally study the stages of thrombosis; it is however, well-accepted that in the early stages of the phenomenon only the platelets take part by adhering to acutely injured vessels. It is because of this reason that the major attention must be given to the behavior of platelets in flowing blood.

The importance of understanding the mechanism of thrombus formation lies not only in the understanding of the phenomenon, but also has much clinical significance. The results of arteriosclerosis and thrombosis are an exceedingly important cause of human morbidity and mortality and a major problem in the use of artificial biomaterial. The most severe manifestations of thrombolic disease are the coronary artery thrombosis leading to myocardial ischemia, thromboembolic occlusion of the cerebral arteries, and venous thrombosis leading to lung embolism. It is important in the development of cardiac and renal transplants, the use of artificial heart valves and vascular grafts, and also in the arteriovenous fistula for renal dialysis.

The mechanisms related to formation of thrombi are a complex interaction between flowing blood constituents, the blood vessel walls, and the flow conditions (more precisely the disturbances to blood flow) which is sometimes defined incorrectly as deviation of blood flow from a laminar pattern.

It is usually asserted that the various components of blood cannot adhere and do not interact with healthy intact endothelium, although the process can be triggered by platelets adhering to collagen or collagen-like materials in the gaps between healthy endothelial cells. When the endothelial structures are exposed to the flowing blood, platelets start to adhere to the subendothelial structures in a matter of milliseconds. This may be different in exposure of blood to artificial material, as different material with different thrombogenic properties trigger different mechanisms and stimulate the accumulation of different blood constituents.

B. Mechanisms in the Different Stages of Thrombus Formation

The process of thrombus formation within the arterial system begins by various mechanisms that trigger platelet reactions. The initial stage consists of a mass of platelet aggregates that adhere to the surface of injured endothelium. This initiation stage usually follows changes of the inner surface of the vessel wall that take only a few seconds. This change is associated with the exposure of subendothelial fibers that include the basement membrane, microfibrils associated with elastin and collagen to the flowing blood. The platelets react with these materials within a few seconds, Chandler.[7] The adhering of the platelets to the injured endothelium involves two concurrent phenomena: the platelets lose their discoid shape while they spread out over the surface of the vessel wall and the release of their granule constituent, of which ADP (adenosine phosphase) is the most important in the formation of aggregate. It is yet to be known what the triggering mechanisms for these two reactions are and what the influence of one on the other is. It is, however, known that ADP released from platelets plays a major role in the aggregation. On the other hand, the increased tendency to form aggregates is due also to the change in size and shape which results in increased volume and a decrease in surface potential.[15] Further developments of the formation of thrombi depend on the flow conditions, the supply of platelets, and the existence of other blood constituents near the adhering platelets. Further platelet aggregation usually takes place together with formation of fibrin around the growing mass. Extensive fibrin formation, mainly when associated with diminished or altered blood flow, activates the coagulation mechanism which can trap flowing red blood cells. This process may eventually lead to occlusion of the vessel lumen. This mechanism is a defense mechanism to arrest capillary bleeding, yet in the same time might be very dangerous to the entire circulation. During the development of this first stage, fragments of the thrombus may break off and pass into the flowing blood to the distal parts of the circulation. It is thus possible to determine the termination stage of thrombus formation (the end of thrombus growth) which can come either because the vessel lumen is occluded or because the formed plug is detached by the bloodstream and moves along into the distal circulation. In the first case, further coagulation of the blood distal and proximal to the site of occlusion might take place within minutes after the initial stage. This is more apt to happen in bedridden patients, especially in postoperative cases.

Copley[9] suggested a new theory on the initiation and growth mechanism. According to his concept, the process of thrombus formation begins with the absorption of fibrinogen followed by layer-by-layer growth of fibrinogen and other plasma proteins. It is only after the vessel lumen is partially or completely obstructed that the aggregation of platelets and red blood cells occurs. In this theory the process that initiates thrombosis occurs in a plasmatic zone near the vessel wall. This zone according to Copley and King is cell-free.[10]

It can be summarized that five important mechanisms are operating in this sequence of events:

1. The interaction of platelets with the endothelial and subendothelial structures of the vessel wall
2. The release of ADP and the formation of thrombin that affect the surface potential and the shape of the platelets
3. The adherence of platelets to nonplatelet surfaces
4. The adherence of platelets to each other
5. The flow conditions of blood

This chapter is devoted to the fluid mechanic aspects of thrombus formation. For further reading of the biochemistry of thrombosis the reader is referred to Jorgensen,[18] Surgenor,[24] Haust,[17] Mustard,[20] Pareti and Capitanio,[21] and other sources.

C. Hemodynamic Factors in Thrombus Formation

A considerable effort has been applied in the last two decades toward the understanding of the biochemistry and physiology of thrombus formation. It is also known that fluid flow plays a highly significant role in atherogenesis and thrombus formation, and that the thrombus structure, shape and size depend on the local blood flow conditions. However, the physical factors associated with disturbed flow and their influence on the initiation of thrombosis are not well understood. Thrombus formation has been supposed to be intimately related to retarded blood flow ("stasis"). This is mainly due to the high incidents of venous thrombosis and the poor performance of artificial biomaterial implants in veins, and to the observations of selective thrombi growth in regions of stagnation or very low flows. However, as pointed out by Roach[23] stasis alone does not initiate thrombosis, as in the case of the umbilical artery where flow stops completely yet the blood remains in a liquid state for a few days after the flow is ceased. On the other hand, thrombus might form in arteries even with strong flow. It is therefore important to discuss a variety of hemodynamic factors that are probable triggering mechanisms in the initiation of thrombosis. These phenomena include deviations from the normal blood flow conditions and are defined as flow disturbances. Table 1 lists the different flow disturbances and the most probable mechanism associated with each of them, however, it should be made clear that all of these phenomena might be interrelated or lead to one another by different thrombogenic reactions.

Stasis results in a regional stagnant flow causing coagulation of blood at the stagnation. Although the mechanism here is different from the regular thrombosis it will continue in a much similar fashion by adhering of platelets to the nonendothelial surface that is formed followed by trapping other blood constituents that flow by and thus leading to reinforcement of the plug causing termination of flow in the vessel.

Different mechanisms are taking place in regions of low velocity. Such regions of retarded flow can result from geometrical reasons such as vessel aneurysms or from separation of the boundary layer or the formation of vortices. In a flow with low velocity profile the collision of platelets with each other or the collision of red blood cells have much higher probability of sticking to each other for longer periods of time, a phenomenon associated with the release of ADP, thus causing the formation of aggregates in the flowing blood, as shown in Table 1. Additional contribution to platelet aggregation in these types of flow is the increased diffusion of platelets and red blood cells. The flow of blood under normal conditions can be considered as a convective diffusion process with convection being the dominant mechanism. When flow velocity is decreased the flow tends to be that of diffusion-controlled flow which, as will be shown later, is leading to a diffusion-controlled thrombus formation.

Local flow disturbances, such as vortices, turbulence, or low pressure in a vicinity or constriction that leads to a formation of gas bubbles known as cavitation, may influence the formation of thrombi by collisions with the vessel walls causing injury to the endothelial layer. The endothelial damage which results in exposure of subendothelial structures to the flowing blood is an immediate site for thrombus formation.

Shear stress has been a controversial subject in relation to its contribution to atherogenesis. On one hand higher shear rates might result in endothelial damage triggering adhering of platelets to the vessel wall, yet on the other hand preventing larger aggregates from forming at these high shear locations. In the very same way low shear near the vessel wall will keep the endothelium intact yet change the mass transfer mechanism. This subject as well as the influence of other blood disturbances will be analyzed in the following sections.

D. Theory of Coagulation

The interaction of the different blood constituents with one another, known as the process of coagulation, is due to a sequence of mechanical and chemical events. The

Table 1

SEQUENCE OF EVENTS THAT RESULT FROM CONDITIONS OF DISTURBED FLOW

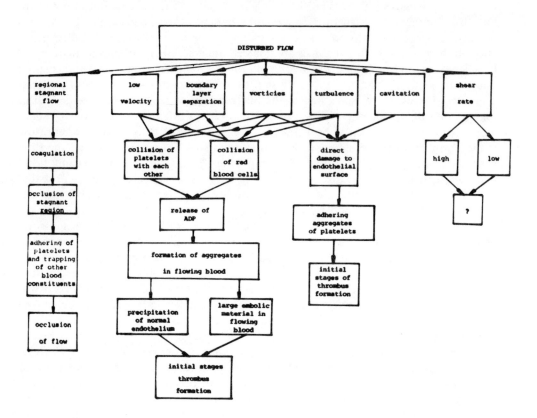

initiation of the process, although different in different chemical environments, is due to hydrodynamic reactions that result from flow conditions, body forces, Brownian motion, and the repulsion force that exists due to electric charge on the outer surface of the different particles. It is thus expected that a different reaction will take place under different flow conditions. In the case of stagnant flow the particles encounter each other solely due to Brownian motion, while in the case of sedimentation there is interaction of the Brownian and gravitational motions. This is mainly due to increased particle concentration in the lower layers of the blood sample used in the sedimentation tests. The more complex phenomenon is the coagulation process in flowing blood which is closely related to a convective diffusion mechanism. It is, however, necessary to consider the simple case of stagnant coagulation prior to attempting the more complex relations of convective diffusion. The analysis of blood coagulation due to Brownian motion must be considered separately for particles of different average size and different geometries. Hence, three different interactions are of importance: platelet-platelet, RBC-RBC, and interactions between platelets and red blood cells. The major contribution to interaction comes from collisions among the various particles, though not every collision results in bonding of the species to a larger aggregate. Levich[19] distinguished between "rapid coagulation", where bonding occurs at each collision and "slow collision", which takes place when stabilizing factors are present in the solution.

The theory of rapid coagulation was developed by Smoluchowski[27] for low concentration of particles and the assumption that encounters between particles occurs only in pairs. Under this assumption the concentration, C, of specific particle is given by:

$$\frac{\partial c}{\partial t} = D \frac{1}{r^2} \frac{\partial}{\partial r}\left(r^2 \frac{\partial c}{\partial r}\right) \tag{1}$$

where D is the Brownian diffusion coefficient. The initial and boundary condition are taken at the outer radius of an assumed sphere of influence, where particles are actually attracted to each other, which for the case of equal size particles is equal to 2a, and at infinity. This is given by:

$$c = c_0 \quad \text{for} \quad r > 2a, \quad t = 0$$

$$c = 0 \quad \text{at} \quad r = 2a, \quad t > 0 \tag{2}$$

$$c = c_0 \quad \text{at} \quad r \to \infty, \quad t > 0$$

where c_0 is the average concentration of the specific specie in the blood plasma. A solution to the last equation satisfying the given conditions yields the following flux of particles arriving at the surface of a given particle per unit time.

$$N^\star = 16 \pi a c_0 D \left[1 + \frac{a}{\sqrt{\pi D t}}\right] \tag{3}$$

which can be approximated by the leading term only, thus eliminating the time dependency of the solution. The Brownian diffusion coefficient can be replaced by the Stokes-Einstein relation:

$$D = \frac{kT}{6\pi\mu a} \tag{4}$$

where T is the absolute temperature and k is the Boltzmann constant. Inserting this value into Equation 3 yields:

$$N_B^\star = \frac{8kT}{3\mu} C_0 \tag{5}$$

As this is the number of collisions for a single particle, the total number of collisions is given by:

$$N_B = \frac{8kT}{3\mu} C_0{}^2 \tag{6}$$

For particles of different radii a_1 and a_2 and with different concentrations C_1 and C_2 this equation is given by:

$$N_B = \frac{2kT}{3\mu} (a_1 + a_2)\left(\frac{1}{a_1} + \frac{1}{a_2}\right) C_1 C_2 \tag{7}$$

Although this equation is good for very small concentrations it is most commonly used as a good approximation for the total number of collisions due to Brownian motion in normal human blood. To obtain the relation for slow coagulation the equation is multiplied by an efficiency factor that accounts for the fact that not each collision results in adhesion of the two colliding particles. The efficiency factor is related to the release reaction of ADP and thrombin and to the destruction of the surface zeta potential.

In the case of laminar flow there are additional collisions due to different velocities of particles with different distances from the vessel walls. To obtain a comparison between collisions due to Brownian motion and those resulting from laminar flow consider the latter case by itself disregarding the effect of Brownian motion. This type of coagulation which takes place because of the existence of velocity gradient is defined as the gradient coagulation. If a particle moves along a pathway at a distance r from the wall, there is another particle at a distance r + Δr moving with a higher velocity. For simplicity the first particle can be considered at rest, thus referencing all velocities to his velocities. The other particle has in this case a velocity which is given by:

$$V_z(\Delta r) = \frac{\partial V_z}{\partial r} \Delta r = G\Delta r \tag{8}$$

where G is the velocity gradient of the flowing blood. If the distance between the trajectories of the two particles is less than the sum of the two radii, the particles will collide after sufficient time to overcome the longitudinal distance between the particles. Assuming an imaginary sphere equal to the "collision" distance, which is twice the diameter of a particle for a collision of equal sized particles, and integrating the particles that are likely to cross this sphere during a specified period, yields the following relations for the total number of collisions in this specified time:

$$N_c = \frac{32}{3} C_0^2 G(2a)^3 = \frac{256}{3} GC_0^2 a^3 \tag{9}$$

for particles of equal size, and:

$$N_c = \frac{32}{3} G(a_1 + a_2)^3 C_1 C_2 \tag{10}$$

for particles of different sizes, a_1 and a_2 are the appropriate radii, and different concentration C_1 and C_2.

The relative importance of these two mechanisms can be evaluated by the ratio of particle collisions under these two conditions:

$$\frac{N_c}{N_B} = \frac{16G a_1 a_2 (a_1 + a_2)}{kT} \tag{11}$$

The interpretation of this equation is that the relative importance of the Brownian and shear type collisions is determined by the rate of shear and the size of the colliding particles. When this ratio is very small, the Brownian motion is the main contributor to coagulation, while at high values of this ratio (e.g., large shear rates) the gradient coagulation is predominant. It should be noted that to obtain upper and lower bonds for aggregation of different blood constituents, it is necessary to include in this ratio the efficiency of the two types of collision. However, not much is known about this subject, but in general it is agreed that the efficiency of coagulation in the gradient coagulation case is shear dependent.

These equations describe the collision frequency of a particle with a specific size. To obtain the rate of aggregation the time rate of change of concentration for particles of different sizes must be considered together with the efficiency of collision, which is different for different blood constituents. If α_{nm} is the efficiency of collision between particle n and particle m, the time rate of change of the concentration of particle n in the solution, is given by:

for Brownian motion:

$$\frac{dC_n}{dt} = \frac{kT}{3\mu} \sum_{k=1}^{n-1} \alpha_{nk}^B C_k C_{n-k} (r_k + r_{n-k}) \left(\frac{1}{r_k} + \frac{1}{r_{n-k}} \right)$$

$$- \frac{2kT}{3\mu} C_n \sum_{k=1}^{\infty} \alpha_{nk}^B C_k (r_n + r_k) \left(\frac{1}{r_n} + \frac{1}{r_k} \right) \tag{12}$$

where $\alpha^B{}_{nk}$ represents the efficiency factor for Brownian motion.

For the gradient coagulation case:

$$\frac{dC_n}{dt} = \frac{2G}{3} \sum_{k=1}^{n-1} \alpha_{nk}^c C_k C_{n-k} (r_n + r_{n-k})^3$$

$$- \frac{4}{3} G C_n \sum_{k=1}^{\infty} \alpha_{nk}^c C_k (r_n + r_k)^3 \tag{13}$$

where $\alpha^c{}_{nk}$ describes the efficiency factor for convective diffusion alone.

For all blood constituents it is possible to use the simplification suggested by Smolchowski:

$$(r_i + r_j) \left(\frac{1}{r_i} + \frac{1}{r_j} \right) \simeq 4 \tag{14}$$

The combined time rate of change of concentration for laminar flow is given by addition of the two effects, thus giving:

$$\frac{dC_n}{dt} = \frac{2G}{3} \left\{ \sum_{k=1}^{n} \alpha_{nk}^c C_k C_{n-k} (r_k + r_{n-k})^3 \right.$$

$$- 2C_n \sum_{k=1}^{n} \alpha_{nk}^c C_k (r_n + r_k)^3$$

$$+ \frac{4kT}{3\mu} \sum_{k=1}^{n} \alpha_{nk}^B C_k C_{n-k} \tag{15}$$

$$\left. - 2C_n \sum_{k=1}^{\infty} \alpha_{nk}^B C_k \right\}$$

The first terms inside the parentheses represent the number of particles which result in a particle of size n by coagulation of smaller particles, and the second terms inside the parentheses represent the number of particles of size n which coagulate with other particles. If platelets are assumed to be the smallest particles, Equation 15 can be used to describe the time rate of change of platelet concentration.

$$\frac{1}{C_p} \frac{dC_p}{d\tau} = -\sum_{k=1}^{\infty} \left[1 + K(1 + \rho)^3 \right] C_k \qquad (16)$$

Where the nondimensional groups are defined as:

$$\tau = \frac{8kT}{3\mu} \alpha B ; \quad \rho = \frac{r_k}{r_p} ; \quad K = \frac{\mu Ga^3}{2kT} \frac{\alpha^c}{\alpha B} \qquad (17)$$

An additional assumption of uniform efficiency for all types of collisions for the same type of motion has been introduced.

From Equation 16 it is possible to conclude that the rate of change of platelet concentration will behave as a decaying exponential, thus yielding an exponential rate of growth of platelet aggregate. It can be observed that for sufficiently high value of K the contribution of collisions due to Brownian motion can be neglected. Chang and Robertson[8] obtained similar results for platelet aggregation in a solution composed of platelets alone where the higher size particles are taken as doublets, triplets, etc. obtained by platelet collision (Figure 1). However, a straightforward solution of Equation 16 is not possible since C_k (# C_p) must be calculated by Equation 15, where the value of k takes into consideration multiple aggregates of platelets and single and multiple aggregates of red and white blood cells as well as coagulants resulting from collision of different size particles. Under these conditions the assumption of uniform efficiency factor is no longer true.

In the case of turbulent flow there is a higher mixing of the particles as they move with the turbulent eddy. This will increase substantially the number of encounters and if the diffusion coefficient is assumed to behave in the same way as in the case of laminar flow, its value must be substantially higher. It is therefore possible to assume that turbulence will increase substantially the time rate of coagulation (see Levich[19] and Delichatsios and Probstein[11]).

E. Species Transport to Arterial Wall in Laminar Flow

The most favorable sites for the development of thrombus and atheroma are constrictions, arterial branches and bends, aneurysms, and other regions where separation of flow is known to take place. In these regions the main phenomenon is limited to a thin boundary layer adjacent to the blood vessel wall, while the net flow through the region is relatively unchanged during the initial stages of aggregation. It is, therefore, the conditions of the disturbed flow in the region that will determine the site, size, and the extent of the formation of atheroma or thrombus. The disturbed flow can effect the thrombus formation in two ways which has led to different hypotheses in regard to the shearing effect of the flow. Fry[13,14] has shown that deposition of blood species takes place at regions with very high shear stresses on the endothelial layer. In these cases, as in the case where blood cells are thrown against the endothelium surface, an injury to the endothelial surface exposes the underlying collagen and subendothelial layers and thus initiating platelet aggregation at these sites. The rate of growth for these cases, depends on the number of platelets which arrive and adhere to the damaged vessel wall, as discussed in the previous section. On the other hand, Caro et al.[5,6]

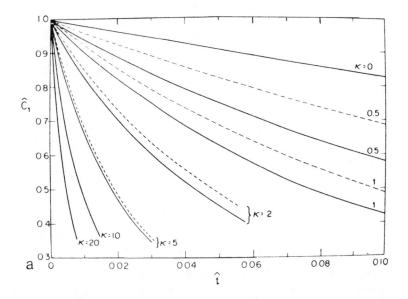

FIGURE 1. Dimensionless multiplet concentration during aggregation. Dashed line — shear motion only. Solid line — shear and Brownian motion. (From Chang, H. N. and Robertson, C. R., *Ann. Biomed. Eng.*, 4, 161, 1976. With permission.)

showed that early atheroma is observed in regions of low shear rates. In this case the mechanism that controls the formation of thrombus, or atheroma, must be different from the injury of the vessel wall. The explanation for this phenomenon might be associated with the porous nature of the endothelial lining and the transport of species through the wall, known as filtration.[1-3] The filtration velocity, which is normal to the wall, determines under these conditions the arrival rate of particles at the site of thrombus formation. The phenomenon which takes place at the site of such disturbed flow is that of boundary layer suction with two distinct boundary layers of flow and particle concentration. For mathematical simplicity, both will be assumed infinite with a stretched radial coordinate, however, they are very small compared to the diameter of the blood vessel. The phenomenon, as will be shown, depends very strongly on the ratio between viscosity and diffusivity expressed by the Schmidt number:

$$S_c = \frac{\nu}{D} \tag{18}$$

In considering the species concentration a different set of equations must be established for each specie. But, it is simpler to consider one specie and to expand the analytical procedure to any desired number of different species. This process necessitates the assumption of linearity or the assumption that there are no interactions among the various species.

In any of the flow regions shown in Figures 2 through 7, the flow is axisymmetric and the equation of mass conservation is given by:

$$\frac{\partial}{\partial x}(ru) + r\frac{\partial v}{\partial y} = 0 \tag{19}$$

where u and v are the parallel and normal velocity components in the directions of x and y, respectively, and r is the radius of the vessel wall which depends only on the

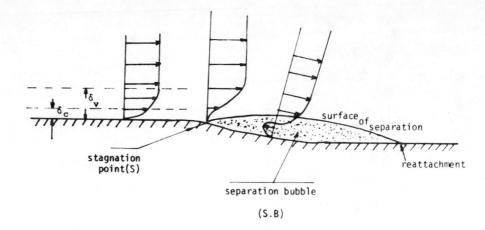

(S.B)

FIGURE 2.   Velocity and concentration boundary layers, showing the surface of separation and stagnation and reattachment points for the velocity in steady laminar flow. δ_v — thickness of velocity boundary layer. δ_c — thickness of concentration boundary layer.

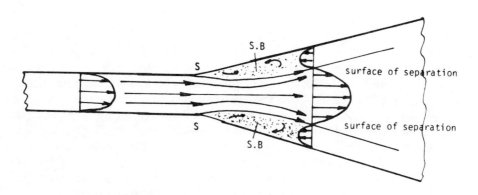

FIGURE 3.   Boundary layer separation at aneurysm, showing velocity distribution and streamlines.

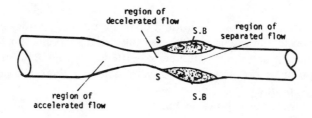

FIGURE 4.   Separation bubble formation is arterial flow past a constriction followed by aneurysm.

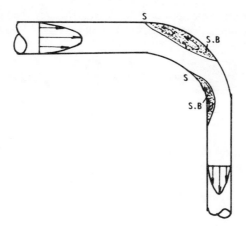

FIGURE 5. Boundary layer separations at bends.

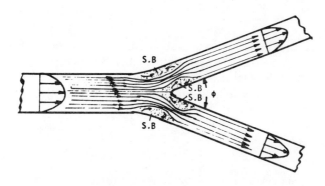

FIGURE 6. Velocity distribution, streamlines and separation bubbles for steady laminar flow in a bifurcation.

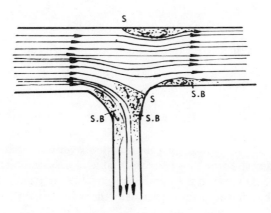

FIGURE 7. Streamlines and separation bubbles for steady laminar flow through a branched artery.

longitudinal coordinate x. The boundary layer equation for the momentum and species mass fraction (weight concentration) C_i are given by:

$$u \frac{\partial u}{\partial x} + \frac{\partial u}{\partial y} = -\frac{1}{\rho} \frac{dP}{dx} + \frac{1}{\rho} \frac{\partial}{\partial y} \left(\mu \frac{\partial u}{\partial y} \right) \qquad (20)$$

$$u \frac{\partial C_i}{\partial x} + \frac{\partial C_i}{\partial y} = \frac{1}{\rho} \frac{\partial}{\partial y} (-\rho_i V_i) \qquad (21)$$

where V_i is the diffusion velocity normal to the wall which is related to the diffusion coefficient by Fick's law:

$$\rho_i V_i = -\rho D_i \frac{\partial C_i}{\partial y} \qquad (22)$$

where ϱ_i is the species density and ϱ is the fluid density. Equation 21 can now be written, assuming that the fluid density is uniform, as:

$$u \frac{\partial C_i}{\partial x} + v \frac{\partial C_i}{\partial y} = \frac{\partial}{\partial y} \left(D_i \frac{\partial C_i}{\partial y} \right) \qquad (23)$$

In writing these equations the longitudinal curvatures of the vessel wall were neglected, as will be done for the application of the boundary conditions. Boundary conditions for the boundary layer equations must apply at the limits of both boundary layers, referred to as the freestream, both velocity and specie mass fraction must approach the values at the freestream namely:

$$u \rightarrow u_e ; \quad C_i \rightarrow C_{ie} \qquad (24)$$

where the subscript e denotes that the value is calculated at the edge of the boundary layer. At the surface of the vessel there is a no-slip condition for the longitudinal velocity component, while the radial (perpendicular) flow must be equal to the filtrate velocity $(-v_w)$:

$$u = 0 ; \quad v = -v_w \qquad \text{at endothelial} \qquad (25)$$

The relations between the arrival rate of particles by diffusion and the filtrate velocity yield:

$$C_i(-v_w) = -D_i \frac{\partial C_i}{\partial y} \qquad \text{at the wall} \qquad (26)$$

The left-hand side has to include only the fraction of species that do not pass into the vessel wall. In reality the number of species that actually penetrate through the porous wall is very small compared to the number of particles arriving at the surface or compared to the number density of particles near the wall that this fraction can be taken as unity.

The method of solution described below is based on the method suggested by Back.[1-3] The nature of the boundary layer equations suggests the existence of a stream function Ψ such that:

$$u = \frac{1}{r} \frac{\partial \Psi}{\partial y} \qquad v = -\frac{1}{r} \frac{\partial \Psi}{\partial x} \tag{27}$$

so that the continuity equation is satisfied. Such a stream function is given by:

$$\Psi = \frac{\sqrt{2\xi}}{\rho} f(\xi, \eta) \tag{28}$$

where ξ and η are new coordinates defined as follows:

$$\xi = \rho \mu_e \int_0^x u_e r^2 dx = \xi(x) \tag{29}$$

$$\eta = \frac{\rho u_e r}{\sqrt{2\xi}} y = \eta(x,y) \tag{30}$$

The velocity is allowed to vary across the boundary layer as a function of species concentration, approaching its freestream value μ_e. The velocities are given in the new coordinate system by:

$$u = u_e \frac{\partial f}{\partial \eta} \tag{31a}$$

$$v = -\frac{\mu_e u_e r}{\sqrt{2\xi}} f - \mu_e u_e r \sqrt{2\xi} \frac{\partial f}{\partial \xi}$$

$$+ \eta \frac{\partial f}{\partial \eta} \left(\frac{\mu_e u_e r}{2\xi} - u_e r \sqrt{2\xi} \frac{du_e}{d\xi} - \mu_e u_e \sqrt{2\xi} \frac{dr}{d\xi} \right) \tag{31b}$$

For simplicity $\partial f/\partial \eta$ will be replaced by f^1. With these results the x momentum equation is transferred to:

$$\left(\frac{\mu}{\mu_e} f^{11} \right)^1 + ff^{11} + \frac{2\xi}{u_e} \frac{du_e}{d\xi} \left[1 - (f^1)^2 \right]$$

$$= 2\xi \left[f^1 \frac{\partial f^1}{\partial \xi} - f^{11} \frac{\partial f}{\partial \xi} \right] \tag{32}$$

Define
$$\beta = \frac{2\xi}{u_e} \frac{du_e}{d\xi} \tag{33}$$

This function is determined by the freestream velocity gradient which in turn depends upon the shape of the vessel wall at the disturbed flow region. In a similar way to the result obtained in Equation 31a, the following expression is considered for the specie concentration:

$$C_i = C_{ie} g(\xi,\eta) \tag{34}$$

which reduces the specie mass traction equation to:

$$\left(\frac{g^1}{S_c}\right)^1 + fg^1 = 2\xi\left[f^1\frac{\partial g}{\partial \xi} - g^1\frac{\partial f}{\partial \xi}\right] \tag{35}$$

Transformation of the boundary conditions give:

$$f^1 \to 1 \; ; \qquad g \to 1 \qquad @ \qquad \eta \to \infty \tag{36a}$$

$$f^1_w = 0$$

$$\left.f_w + 2\xi\left(\frac{\partial f}{\partial \xi}\right)_w = \frac{(-v_w)\sqrt{2\xi}}{\mu_e u_e r}\right\} \tag{36b}$$

$$g_w = -\alpha_w g^1_w$$

where the subscript w denotes the value is taken at the wall, or at $\eta = 0$, and α is a nondimensional parameter defined by:

$$\alpha = \frac{D_i \rho u_e r}{(-v_w)\sqrt{2\xi}} \tag{37}$$

A general solution of Equations 32 and 35 subject to the boundary conditions (Equation 36) is possible only in a numerical way. It is, however, possible to obtain similarity solutions for these equations when ξ is chosen in such a way that β, f_w and α are independent of ξ, and the variable η becomes the similarity variable. The requirement for β independent of ξ determines a relation between u_e and ϱ. This relation through the definition of ξ, Equation 29, defines a class of possible geometries by specification of r as a function of x, or as a function of ξ.

Under conditions of similarity, the species mass fraction equation, 35, is reduced for a constant Schmidt number to:

$$g^{11} + S_c fg^1 = 0 \tag{38}$$

with boundary conditions:

$$g^1 \to 1 \quad \text{at} \quad \eta \to \infty$$

$$g_w = -\alpha g^1_w \quad \text{at} \quad \eta = 0 \tag{39}$$

Integration of this equation gives:

$$g = A\int_0^\eta \exp\left[-\int_0^{\eta_1} S_c f d\eta_1\right] d\eta_1 + B \tag{40}$$

where A and B are constants to be determined by the boundary conditions. The integral

$$I(\eta) = \int_0^\eta \exp\left[-\int_0^{\eta_2} S_c f d\eta_1\right] d\eta_2 \tag{41}$$

is the η dependence of the specie distribution. Inserting the boundary conditions Equation 39 yields:

$$g(\eta) = g_w + I(\eta) g_w^1 \qquad (42)$$

where

$$g_w = \frac{1}{1 - \dfrac{I\infty}{\alpha_w}} \qquad (43)$$

The value of α_w is calculated from Equation 37 at the wall and $I\infty$ is given by Equation 41 as:

$$I\infty = I(\eta = \infty) = \int_0^\infty \exp\left[-\int_0^{\eta_2} S_c f d\eta_1\right] d\eta_2 \qquad (44)$$

The species mass fraction and concentration profile can be fully determined by this relation after solution of the flow is obtained from the momentum equation. This can be done for the general case, however, further simplifications of the equation can be achieved, for this particular case, by estimations of the order of magnitude of the variable parameters. It is simpler to assume special cases of vessel's geometry and obtain solutions for these cases.

The case corresponding to flow in a converging or diverging tapered tube as well as the flow around a collateral stenosis is that of accelerating or decelerating flow. For these cases the freestream velocity distribution can be described by the Falkner-Skan profile:

$$u_e = ax^m \qquad (45)$$

where $m > 0$ describes accelerating flow and $m < 0$ the decelerating case. For a very small thickness of the boundary layer, compared with tube diameter, the average velocity $\bar{u}$ at a given cross section can be replaced by the freestream velocity at this cross section, thus writing the conservation of mass as:

$$\rho\pi r^2 \bar{u} = \rho\pi r^2 u_e = \rho\pi r^2 ax^m = c_1 = \text{const.} \qquad (46)$$

This equation prescribes the possible geometries which enable the use of similarity solutions. This gives the following relation for the vessel radius:

$$r^2 = \frac{C_1}{\pi\rho ax^m} \qquad (47)$$

which gives, upon insertion into Equations 29 and 33,

$$\xi = \frac{\mu_e}{\pi} C_1 x \qquad (48)$$

$$\beta = 2m \qquad (49)$$

The equations for the flow distribution for this case are reduced to:

$$\left(\frac{\mu}{\mu_e} f''\right)' + ff'' + 2m\left[1 - (f')^2\right] = 0 \tag{50}$$

$$f' \to 1 \quad \text{at} \quad \eta = \infty \tag{51}$$

$$\left.\begin{aligned} f'_w &= 0 \\[1em] f_w &= (-v_w)\sqrt{\frac{2\rho}{a\mu_e}}\; x^{\frac{1}{2}(1-m)} \end{aligned}\right\} \tag{52}$$

$$\alpha = \frac{D}{(-v_w)}\sqrt{\frac{\rho a}{2\mu_e}}\; x^{\frac{1}{2}(m-1)} \tag{53}$$

For a uniform filtrate velocity, as well as for uniform α, the only possible value of m is unity, which corresponds to an artery whose radius is decreasing longitudinally as $1/\sqrt{x}$, or the cross-sectional area is decreasing as $1/x$. The values of f_w and α for this case are:

$$f_w = (-v_w)\sqrt{\frac{2}{av_e}} \tag{54}$$

$$\alpha = \frac{D}{(-v_w)}\sqrt{\frac{a}{2v_e}} = \frac{1}{fS_c} \tag{55}$$

If the viscosity is assumed uniform across the boundary layer the flow distribution is fully determined by f_w, yet the specie mass fraction depends on the entire flow field and the Schmidt number.

Back[2] showed that for blood of normal hematocrit (40%) at 37°C, flowing in a coronary artery ($r_w = 1.5$ mm) with a velocity gradient a = 80 1/sec and flow rate of 50 mℓ/min, the filtration parameter f_w is very small (smaller than 10^{-5}), so that the slope of the nondimensional velocity profile f' is described, for all practical purposes, only by f''_w. This together with the fact that the Schmidt number for all the species of blood is relatively large (in the order of 10^5), permits the assumption of the linear relations:

$$f' = f''_w \eta \tag{56}$$

With this linear assumption and results obtained by Hartree[16] and by Elzy and Sisson,[12] Back[13] showed that the wall concentration of species varies as:

$$(g_w - 1)\alpha\;(f''_{wn})^{1/3} \tag{57}$$

where f''_{wn} corresponds to the value of f''_w in the special case where $f_w = 0$.

Velocity profiles and variation of f''_w with the freestream velocity gradients, were obtained by Back[2,3] and are shown in Figures 8 and 9.

From these figures and Equation 57 the following conclusions can be revealed:

1.   In the case of accelerated flow which corresponds to a converging tapered blood vessel (normal arterial vessel) the effect of filtrate velocity is very small and the

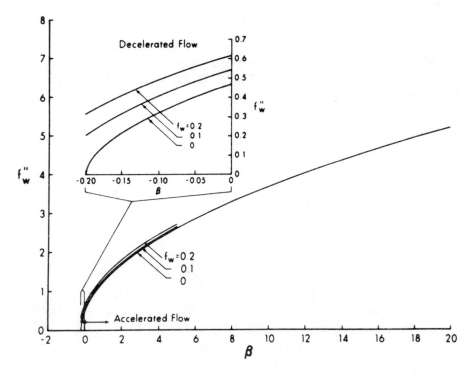

FIGURE 8. Variation of the slope of the velocity profile at the wall, f_w'', with the freestream velocity gradient parameter β. (From Back, L. H., *Math. Biosci.*, 27, 1975. With permission.)

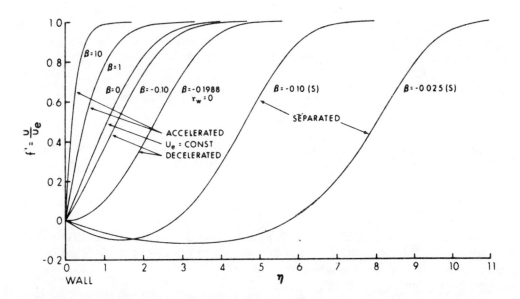

FIGURE 9. Velocity profiles — similarity solutions — $f_w = 0$. Accelerated, decelerated, and separated flows. (From Back, L. H., *Math Biosci.*, 27, 1975. With permission.)

general effect of acceleration is to reduce the number of species that accumulate on the vessel walls.

2. The opposite phenomenon takes place in decelerated flows, which takes place at sites of aneurysm of the vessel or in the distal parts of a constriction. In these cases f^{11}_w decreases and therefore there is an increase in the number of species accumulated at the wall. The excess mass fraction at the wall may serve as a triggering mechanism for the formation of thrombus, even if the endothelial layer is intact.

3. Similar excess specie mass fraction occurs in cases of reduced arterial flow and at sites of boundary layer separation.

The shear stress at the wall is given by:

$$\tau_w = \mu_w \left(\frac{\partial u}{\partial y} + \frac{\partial v}{\partial x}\right)_w = \left(\frac{\mu_w}{\mu_e}\right)(\rho\mu_e)^{1/2} a^{3/2} x^{\frac{3m-1}{2}} f^{11}_w \quad (58)$$

so that the shear stress at the wall is linearily proportioned to f^{11}_w. This equation, together with Equation 57, yields a relation between the species mass fraction and shear stress:

$$(g_w - 1)\alpha \, \tau^{-3/2} x^{\frac{3m-1}{6}} = K_1 \tau^{1/3} x^{\frac{3m-1}{6}} \quad (59)$$

where K_1 depends on the physical constants of the system. Considering that species mass fraction at the wall depends linearly on the flux of particles at the wall area that is available for deposition and the efficiency of wall-particles interactions, it is possible to conclude that the flux, J, of particles reaching the wall is equal to:

$$J = K_1^\star \, \tau_w^{1/3} \, x^{-\frac{3m-1}{6}} \quad (60)$$

which for the case $m = 1$ reduces to:

$$J = K_1^\star \left(\frac{\tau_w}{x}\right)^{1/3} \quad (61)$$

This equation is equivalent to the relations obtained by Turitto[25] and Turitto and Baumgartner[26] for deposition of particles on a probe exposed to whole blood in laminar flow, and analyzed by Baumgartner and Muggli.[4] The equation for the flux used by them is given by:

$$J = K_2 \left(\frac{\tau_w D}{x}\right)^{1/3} \quad (62)$$

The factor K_2 depends on the physical parameters of the system but is independent of the physical dimensions of the system. The importance of the use of the diffusivity as a separate parameter can be explained by the experimental results obtained by Turitto and Baumgartner[26] for the platelet coverage of the subendothelial layer. They measured the surface deposition of platelets as a function of time and calculated the best straight line in logarithmic coordinate. The slope which must equal 0.333 according to this theory, was actually much higher, 0.61 ± 0.06, suggesting that the platelet diffusivity depends on the blood shear rate. This is more so in Back's theory as the flux depends not only on the diffusivity but also on the shear parameter as in Equation 45.

This shows that additional research into the nature of species concentration in laminar flow is necessary to obtain the appropriate relations for platelet deposition on the vessel wall, especially in the case of pulsatile flow which is more complex than the theories presented here, and where very little data are available from experimental findings. The same is true for case of turbulence.

REFERENCES

1. Back, L. H., Theoretical investigation of platelet embolus production in atherosclerotic coronary artery, *Math. Biosci.,* 25, 273, 1975.
2. Back, L. H., Theoretical investigation of mass transport to arterial walls in various blood flow regions. I. Flow field and lipoprotein transport, *Math. Biosci.,* 27, 231, 1975.
3. Back, L. H., Theoretical investigation of mass transport to arterial walls in various blood flow regions. II. Oxygen transport and its relationship to lipoprotein accumulation, *Math. Biosci.,* 27, 263, 1975.
4. Baumgartner, H. R. and Muggli, R., Adhesion and aggregation: morphological demonstration and quantitation in vivo and in vitro, in *Platelets in Biology and Pathology,* Gordon, J. L., Ed., Elsevier/North-Holland, Amsterdam, 1976, 22.
5. Caro, C. G., Fitz-Gerald, J. M., and Schroter, R. C., Arterial wall shear and distribution of early atheroma in man, *Nature,* 223, 1159, 1969.
6. Caro, C. G., Fitz-Gerald, J. M., and Schroter, R. C., Atheroma and arterial wall shear observation, correlation and proposal of a shear dependent mass transfer mechanism for atherogenesis, *Proc. R. Soc. London, Ser. B,* 177, 109, 1971.
7. Chandler, A. B., The platelet in thrombus formation, in *The Platelet,* Brinkhous, K. M., Shermer, R. W., and Mostofi, F. K., Eds., Williams & Wilkins, Baltimore, 1971, 183.
8. Chang, H. N. and Robertson, C. R., Platelet aggregation by laminar shear and Brownian motion, *Ann. Biomed. Eng.,* 4, 161, 1976.
9. Copley, A. L., Non-Newtonian behavior of surface layers of human plasma protein systems and a new concept of the initiation of thrombosis, *Biorheology,* 8, 79, 1971.
10. Copley, A. L. and King, R. G., Polymolecular layers of fibrinogen systems and the genesis of thrombosis, *Thromb. Res.,* 8, 393, 1976.
11. Delichatsios, M. A. and Probstein, R. F., Coagulation in turbulent flow: theory and experiment, *J. Colloid Interface Sci.,* 51, 394, 1975.
12. Elzy, E. and Sisson, R. M., Tables of similar solutions to the equations of momentum, heat and mass transfer in laminar boundary layer flow, *Eng. Exp. Stn. Bull., No. 4,* Oregon State University, Corvallis, 1967.
13. Fry, D. M., Acute vascular endothelial changes associated with increased blood velocity gradients, *Circ. Res.,* 22, 165, 1968.
14. Fry, D. M., Certain histological and chemical responses of the vascular interface to acutely induced mechanical stress in the aorta of the dog, *Circ. Res.,* 24, 93, 1969.
15. Hampton, J. R. and Mitchell, J. R. A., Effect of aggregating agents on the electrophoretic mobility of human platelets, *Br. Med. J.,* 1, 1074, 1966.
16. Hartree, D. R., On an equation occurring in Falkner and Skan's approximate treatment of the equations of the boundary layer, *Proc. Cambridge Philos. Soc.,* 33, 223, 1937.
17. Haust, M. D., Platelets, thrombosis and atherosclerosis, in *Platelets, Drugs and Thrombosis, Symp.,* Hamilton, 1972, Karger, Basel, 1975, 94.

18. Jorgensen, L., Mechanisms of thrombosis, *Pathobiol. Annu.*, 1, 139, 1971.
19. Levich, V., Certain problems in the theory of coagulation of dispersions involving liquid and gases, in *Physiochemical Hydrodynamics*, Prentice-Hall, Englewood Cliffs, N. J., 1962, chap. 5.
20. Mustard, J. F., Platelets, drug and thrombosis: the problem, in *Platelets, Drug and Thrombosis, Symp.*, Hamilton, 1972, Karger, Basel, 1975, 1.
21. Pareti, F. I. and Capitanio, A., Biochemistry and metabolism, in *Platelet: A Multidisciplinary Approach*, deGaetano, G. and Garattini, S., Eds., Raven Press, New York, 1978, 35.
22. Paterson, J. C., The pathology of venous thrombi, in *Thrombosis*, Sherry, S., Brinkhaus, K. M., Genton, E., and Stengle, J. M., Eds., Natl. Acad. Sci. U.S.A., 1969, 321.
23. Roach, M. R., Blood flow and thrombosis particularly in aneurysms, in *Thrombosis: Pathogenesis and Clinical Trials*, Int. Congr., Thromb. and Haemost., Vienna, Austria, 1973, 123.
24. Surgenor, D. M., Erythrocytes and blood coagulation, *Thromb. Diath. Haemorrh.*, 32, 247, 1974.
25. Turitto, V. T., Mass transfer in annuli under conditions of laminar flow, *Chem. Eng. Sci.*, 30, 503, 1975.
26. Turitto, V. T. and Baumgartner, H. R., Platelet deposition of subendothelium exposed to flowing blood: mathematical analysis of physical parameters, *Trans. Am. Soc. Artif. Int. Organs*, 21, 593, 1975.
27. Smoluchowski, M. V., Versuch einer mathematischen Theorie der Koagulationkinetic Kolloider Lösungen, *Z. Phys. Chem. (Leipzig)*, 92, 129, 1917.

INDEX

W

Y

Z